Comments on **Beating Depression – the 'at your fingertips' guide** *from readers*

This is a very good, comprehensive book, that is easy to use and follow. The question and answer format works well, covering many of the most commonly asked questions and worries. This is a book that, when read from cover to cover, can provide a comprehensive overview of depression but can also be kept to hand and dipped into whenever the need arises.

Amelia Mustapha, Depression Alliance

The format of the 'frequently asked questions' is really helpful and I wholeheartedly agree with the content of the answers and the easily readable style. As well as being an excellent resource for the consumer, this text will be an excellent resource for the primary care professional who will be asked these questions on a daily basis.

Professor André Tylee, Professor of Primary Care Mental Health, Institute of Psychiatry, King's College London

All you need to know about depression, presented in a clear, concise and readable way.

Ann Dawson, Director, World Health Organisation Office for Quality, Noncommunicable Disease and Conditions

I found the book very informative, well documented, and of great help. All the topics are well covered – the symptoms particularly I could really identify with. I felt all the better for perusing *Beating Depression.*   *J.C., Saffron Walden*

I found the self-help advice particularly useful, and I'm keeping a list of my favourite techniques on my bedside table. I thought there was good advice for everybody – teenagers to grannies – in this book. And I liked that poem.   *R.D., Bath*

A really useful guide for anyone who wants to know more about depression and how to manage it. Something for people of all ages, young and old.

P.H., Senior Clinical Nurse Specialist (Mental Health)

I've found that depression is a complex condition, but the authors have manage͏   reader-friendly. It's not too heav   sweet and easy to understand.   *J.R., Carmarthen*

GW00482570

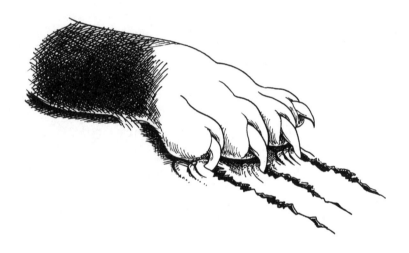

BEATING DEPRESSION

The 'at your fingertips' guide

THE COMPLETE GUIDE TO DEPRESSION AND HOW TO OVERCOME IT

Dr Stefan Cembrowicz MB ChB MRCGP
Senior Partner in General Practice at the Montpelier Health Centre,
Bristol; GP Trainer and Honorary University Teacher;
Member of the Avon Suicide Prevention Group

Dr Dorcas Kingham MRCS LRCP MB ChB MRCPI MRCPsych
Consultant Psychiatrist in General Adult Psychiatry,
Medical Director of the Bristol Priory Hospital

CLASS PUBLISHING • LONDON

Dedication

To our respective partners,
Mary-Jane and Jonathan

© Stefan Cembrowicz, Dorcas Kingham 2002

The rights of Stefan Cembrowicz and Dorcas Kingham to be identified as the authors of this work have been asserted by them in accordance with the Copyright, Designs and Patents Act 1988.

Printing history
First published 2002

The author and the publishers welcome feedback from the users of this book. Please contact the publishers:
Class Publishing (London) Ltd,
Barb House, Barb Mews,
London W6 7PA
Telephone: 0207 371 2119
Fax: 0207 371 2878 [International +44171]

A CIP catalogue record for this book is available from the British Library

ISBN 1 85959 063 2

Edited by Michèle Clarke

Cartoons by William Rankin

Illustrations by David Woodroffe

Indexed by Val Elliston

Typeset by Martin Bristow

Printed and bound in Finland by WS Bookwell, Juva

Contents

Acknowledgements

We should like to thank the following for kindly reviewing and commenting upon the text: Dr Ann Dawson, World Health Organisation; Marjorie Wallace and Ceri-Jane Hackling, Sane; Amelia Mustafa, Depression Alliance; Professor André Tylee, Institute of Psychiatry, King's College London.

We should also like to thank Daniel and Ruth Levy for kindly agreeing to be our cover models.

viii

Foreword

Dr Cembrowicz and Dr Kingham have produced a sympathetic and understanding guide for those people who experience depression. The variations of depression are explained clearly and concisely and the authors give simple explanations about causes and help available.

The book covers a wide range of topics from depression, bipolar disorder and postnatal depression, to alcohol and drugs and how they can affect depression and recovery.

The question and answer sections are invaluable since they focus on patients and the questions families most frequently ask, and respond to them in terms that are easily understood, non-alarmist and compassionate.

Depression is a frightening and lonely illness and the authors offer practical advice on common problems such as how to manage feelings of inadequacy, frustration or despair, whether at home or work, and techniques for living with the symptoms, such as insomnia, agitation, panic and apathy.

Beating Depression – the 'at your fingertips' guide combines medical expertise with a commonsense approach that is neither patronising nor technical. It is an invaluable guide to people suffering from mental illness, their families and friends.

Marjorie Wallace

Chief Executive of SANE

Foreword

It is now over twelve years since the birth of my son, Matthew, which heralded the darkest time of my life – the onset of post-natal depression.

At that time many doctors did not accept it existed and at first I found it difficult to get information and guidance about the illness. I was fortunate to have a loving and supportive family but sadly many do not, as the many letters I have read testify.

Beating Depression would have been a very welcome book at that time as it explains in very clear terms all the different aspects of depression in all its many forms and tries to explain all the whys and wherefores to help all sufferers understand their illness.

Even after twelve years there is still information here that I found interesting and helpful. I wish it every success.

Denise Welch

Introduction

Depression is the commonest illness of all: 40% of the population will experience this condition at some time in their lives. It may be mild or severe. It can be a brief phase in someone's life, or can lead to prolonged personal unhappiness, sometimes even to self-harm or long-term disability. It is often associated with anxiety symptoms.

It occurs with many other physical illnesses, yet may sometimes pass unrecognised by doctors, families and even by people themselves. It can be difficult to recognise particularly when it occurs in childhood, postnatally or in later life.

Families of people with depression may have many concerns and questions about the condition which medical staff may find difficult to answer because of problems of time and issues of confidentiality.

Depression can present in many ways: it can mimic other medical conditions; it can appear associated with fatigue, stress, headaches, poor work or academic performance, marital difficulties, alcohol or drug problems, or for no obvious reason at all. Causes may be deep-seated – or sometimes surprisingly straightforward. It may present quite differently in those from other cultures.

Treatments include the 'talking treatments' (various types of psychotherapy) and medication. Both long-established and newly developed medications are effective, as is at least one alternative herbal remedy. None of these is without some side-effect. General practitioners treat most cases; but people who are more severely depressed may be treated by psychiatrists, in outpatient clinics or as hospital inpatients.

However this illness affects you, a friend, or a member of your family, we hope that you will find something helpful in the following pages. We've used a wide variety of descriptions of depression, its causes and its best treatment, ranging from brain chemistry to social explanations. We have tried to include something for everybody.

1
What is depression?

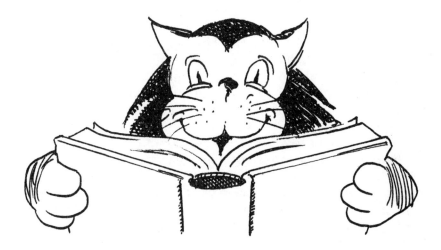

Every human being has changes in their mood. Experiencing good, not so good, and low mood is normal. The variety of our feelings is essential to our being lively and responsive to our surroundings. We would otherwise be totally predictable and robotic. Contrasting moods and feelings add depth to our lives. There will be times when elated, or extra good mood, is appropriate – something really good has happened and we are very happy. It will also be entirely appropriate to feel low, tearful and negative in other circumstances, for example being made redundant. The difference, however, between that experience and being depressed, can be subtle but all important. It is the difference between normal experience and illness. Many people would feel bad at losing a job but not everyone would go on to be ill. Illness begins and normal experience ends, at the point at which your everyday functioning is affected and continues to be affected beyond what would reasonably be expected. You would not expect a person who has lost their livelihood last week to be functioning well this week, but you would expect a gradual improvement over the course of the following months. If this (normal) mood is protracted and it starts to change the way someone is coping (or not coping) with life, it starts to become a problem or illness.

A very helpful definition of depressive illness was given by Sir Aubrey Lewis in the 1950s. He said depressed people are 'sad, and ill with their sadness' – this means not just low mood but, because they are ill, there are changes in the way their bodies are functioning. There can be a whole variety of symptoms, which we shall discuss later in the book, but there are common important changes that happen in clinical depression – or the illness depression. Sleep rhythms can be disrupted, and sleep can deteriorate badly. Depressed people often wake in the early hours of the morning and can't get back to sleep again. Their appetite changes – it usually decreases with loss of weight, although sometimes, and less commonly, appetite increases (comfort eating). Concentration can deteriorate. Memory can be 'fuzzy'. Sexual interest often diminishes. Thoughts can be slowed down. These are all measurable changes and are signs of illness, rather than a simple, well circumscribed period of sadness.

Frequently asked questions about depression

How common is depression?

Depression of one sort or another is the commonest illness of all; it's said that 40% of all of us get this illness at some time in our lives. Nearly a quarter of all GP attendances are for some form of emotional problem; 3% of the population are estimated to be suffering from depression, and 8% suffer from mixed anxiety and depression, at any one time. Many more people, who don't have a full-scale illness, have difficulties or disabilities owing to some depressive symptoms.

There is a wide range of severity of this remarkable illness. It can range from a quite subtle loss of enthusiasm and pleasure in life, which is hardly even recognised by the person concerned or their family, to a severe condition that can need urgent hospital treatment for the patient's safety.

Most cases of depression are in the mild to moderate range. So about 90% of people with depression will be most appropriately treated by their family doctors, generally with a combination of antidepressants and counselling.

The other 10% will need more intensive and specialised looking after by a psychiatrist – and members of their team, such as clinical psychologists, community psychiatric nurses, and other therapists. Only a very small percentage will actually need treatment in hospital. This is relatively quite rare.

Depression can have accumulated over *many* years and a catalyst could have set the final crumple-switch into action, to cause the breakdown to develop into severe depression. Many people do not recognise it happening to them. Others around them can also be blind to it or don't seem able to help.

Will I ever feel better?

Yes. A very common part of depressive illness is feeling negative and having a bleak view of the future. The belief that the illness will go on forever fades as the illness is treated. With treatment, people describe a feeling as if a cloud has lifted, as if the light has been switched back on, or as if the colour has come back into their lives. They often add that they never believed they could or would get better. It takes months for a complete course of treatment, often 6–9 months. You may well feel some benefit after a few days on antidepressants, in terms of sleep pattern starting to improve, and moods in the daytime becoming less variable, but a full course of treatment does require patience.

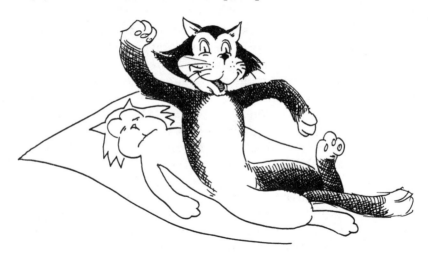

What are the chances of becoming depressed again?

If you have already had a depressive illness you have an increased chance of it happening again – but it is by no means inevitable. The rate is approximately 10 times higher than in somebody who has never been depressed before. If there has been more than one previous episode, the rate is about 15 times higher. This does not, however, mean that the severity of the illness is as great. After experiencing depression, people always learn about their illness – they tend to spot it much earlier and seek treatment earlier. The people around them also tend to be quicker to spot depression developing. Having had a depressive illness, you will have coping strategies that the experience will have taught you. Remember that depression is a very common illness and affects 3% of the population a year. A very large number of those people are functioning both at home and at work, despite being ill.

Will my depression come back?

About 50% of people who have depression never experience it again. The older you are when you become depressed, and the more episodes of depression you have had, the greater is your likelihood of further spells of depression. People who have had several spells of illness may need to consider long-term medication. This sort of decision needs careful thought and advice from a specialist.

What makes relapse more likely?

Risk increases if mood is fairly constantly low or dysthymic – in other words a truly normal mood pattern has not been re-established and your mood remains consistently below par. If there is a concurrent physical illness (especially if painful), the risk of relapse is higher. Relapse of depression is more likely if you are drinking alcohol to excess, or if you have a second psychiatric illness in addition to depression.

Relapse is more likely if difficult and painful problems have not been addressed. The feeling of being trapped in a difficult situation is a very stressful position to be in and increases the chance of further trouble. People can, and do, cope with great adversity. If, however, you feel powerless, and as though you have no choices, then stresses are much greater to bear. We can live in difficult situations, including problematic marriages or a very demanding job, if we feel that we ourselves have made a conscious decision to do this.

Does depression get better on its own?

Yes. Even very severe depressive illness can get better on its own, but there is always the risk in untreated serious depression of death by suicide, or sometimes (especially in the elderly) by self-neglect.

How long does it take to get better?

About half of the people who become depressed will recover within less than 6 months, but about 1 in 10 seriously depressed people may take up to 2 years to recover fully.

Why are some people slow to get better?

This is a complicated question. One of the most important reasons for not getting better is stopping treatment before advised. Fewer than half the people prescribed antidepressants will still be taking them after three months' treatment. They may stop taking the tablets for a variety of reasons, including:

- unacceptable side-effects;
- the fact that they are feeling better;
- pressures from family members to stop taking tablets, or
- fear that antidepressants are addictive (they aren't!).

Remember to tell your doctor if you have stopped taking the tablets prescribed – he or she needs to know. Otherwise the doctor might think that you are not responding to the tablets rather than the fact that you are not taking them. Not all tablets will work in everyone. A quarter of depressed people will respond to the first antidepressant that the GP prescribes. You cannot tell by just looking at someone which type of anti-depressant will suit that particular person best. Overall about 60% of depressed people will respond to an antidepressant taken in adequate doses for an adequate length of time.

Our daughter developed severe depression as a teenager. We can't help feeling it's our fault. Could we be to blame?

It is always painful to see a loved one depressed – particularly so a child or adolescent. There is often a tendency in parents to blame themselves and believe that any professionals involved in trying to treat will be critical of parents. Professional help is not about blaming but enabling people to deal with their difficulties in a different way. Most children and adolescents who become depressed will get better with time and care (both of which parents can provide). Expert intervention will also help and a wide range of agencies are used for this, including health visitors, child guidance clinics, educational psychologists, nurses, social workers and doctors, as well as resources from the voluntary sector and churches.

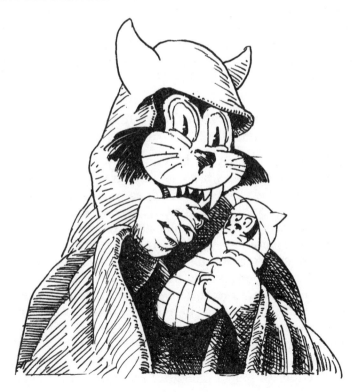

Can you be depressed and not realise it? Looking back on my life I see that there were spells of time when I switched off from things and stagnated. I wasn't happy or unhappy, but I just couldn't take much interest in anything. I let things slide – my job, my social life, even my appearance. Would you call this depression?

It probably was, although hindsight is a wonderful thing. Few people's moods are constant, level and settled; some people do have times in their lives when their enjoyment of life may wax and wane. There is a fine line between unhappiness and mild to moderate depressive illness. Loneliness and boredom at some stages are routine experiences for many people, but when you lose the ability to do something about your life, take charge of things and make some good changes so that you are no longer lonely and bored, then illness may be appearing.

Broken sleep with early morning wakening, loss of appetite and sex drive, mood swings, loss of insight and concentration, and loss of pleasure in life are signs of illness, as opposed to just plain misery.

Some of my family members have had depression. Does this mean I'm going to wind up like them?

The late Anthony Storr, psychiatrist and writer, has said, 'It's not your psychopathology, it's what you do with it that counts.' What he meant was that we all have a set of personality characteristics, some influenced by our inherited genes, but *nothing is inevitable*, and everybody has choices in how they use their own personality and character – for better or worse. Of course, we all have a mixture of strengths and weaknesses in our personalities. If you do have a family tendency towards depression or alcoholism, it does not mean that your life is going to be over-whelmed by these illnesses. It does mean, however, that you may face more emotional challenges, be more vulnerable than some other people, and that you will have to face up to looking after yourself carefully in this particular area. Having good friends around you is a great help. Remember, nothing is inevitable.

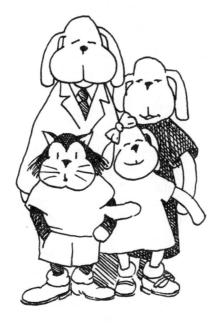

Types of depression

Whole textbooks are written about the classification of different types of depression. The terminology can be very confusing. Some of the headings that have been used include:

Primary and secondary depression

Primary depression means the illness has developed on its own. Secondary depression means the depression has been caused by another illness – the depression is a complication of another medical problem such as the thyroid gland over- or under-working, or as a result of taking certain medications. Medicines that can contribute to depression include steroids, and some of the antihypertensive drugs (given for high blood pressure). Alcohol, our favourite drug, is a strong depressor of mood and, if used in excess, depression can occur. Depression would then be secondary – or follow from alcohol abuse. There are many other causes.

Neurotic depression and psychotic depression

So-called neurotic depression has an unfortunate name. What it actually means is that the depressed person is, no matter how ill they are, always in touch with reality. This makes an important distinction between neurotic depression and psychotic depression. A psychotic person loses touch with reality (and this may be in one small area only), or their beliefs may be wide ranging in their abnormality. People can become psychotic in the setting of many types of mental illness – not only some types of depression.

People suffering from psychotic illnesses have delusions. This means that the person has a fixed false belief which is not in keeping with the generally accepted beliefs of their culture. If I said that I believe the world is flat, I would be deluded – we know the world is not flat – but had I lived at the time of Socrates and said the world was flat, I would not have been deluded but just expressing a piece of current, ancient Greek knowledge. Delusions in illnesses usually have far more significance than this and can cause great suffering. If, for instance, you believe that the water supply is being poisoned by your neighbour, you will be very frightened and you will stop drinking.

Endogenous and exogenous depression

This terminology is little used now and is probably not that helpful. Endogenous depression refers to a depressive illness that comes (from within) – it happens with no obvious cause. Exogenous depression refers to the sort of depression that happens as a response to a stressful event, like a divorce, or a bereavement – it had an outside 'cause'. There was a life-event, or happening that caused the depression. This may at first seem persuasive but, in fact, if you look at any group of depressed people they are *all* more likely to have big things (life-events) happening in their lives in the 2 years before their illness developed, compared with people who are currently well. If you are ill with depression, you will respond to treatment in the same way whether or not your illness is 'explainable'. It makes no difference.

Unipolar and bipolar affective disorder (or manic-depressive disorder)

About 1 in 10 people with depression will have a manic-depressive illness, also called *bipolar affective disorder*. Besides spells of low mood and depression, they will experience mood swings in the other direction. In severe cases, psychotic features can occur.

These are very important and useful ways of describing depressive illness. Unipolar depression means a depressive illness that has happened in a person who is either experiencing normal mood, or is depressed. These are the states that they feel, the mood does not swing further. Somebody with bipolar illness on the other hand, characteristically experiences normal, depressed, and 'high' or elated moods at different times. Their mood swings between normal, too bright, and too low – they experience the two poles of mood experience. They visit both ends of the spectrum of mood – very up and very down – and this can be extremely incapacitating. It is important to make the distinction because people with manic-depressive illness respond better to a different set of treatments than people who become 'only' or solely depressed.

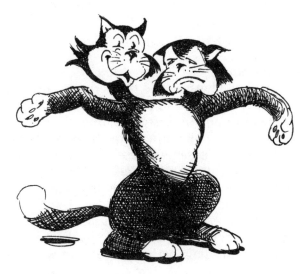

The two types of illnesses – unipolar and bipolar illness – are different in other important ways. For example, if you are bipolar (or manic-depressive), you are more likely to have a family member who is similarly ill than if you have a unipolar depressive illness.

My mum has manic-depressive (bipolar) disorder. What are the chances of my getting it, or of my children having it?

About 1% of the population will develop bipolar disorder, so it is much less common than ordinary depression. If a close relative (your parent, brother or sister) has bipolar illness, then your chances are greater, but probably still only about 20%, of having some kind of mood disorder and it may be less severe. It is still relatively unlikely to happen to you.

Rather than worrying about whether you will develop the same condition, perhaps the best advice is to 'know yourself' and be aware of what your moods are like. Then recognise and manage stressful situations that could unsettle you, as we shall describe in future chapters.

The relatives of people with bipolar disorder are often more creative and successful than the average, so having these genes somewhere in your family can sometimes have good side-effects.

How doctors classify mental illness

ICD10 is the *International Classification of Disease*. It is a way of classifying mental illnesses and is internationally understood and accepted. This makes the diagnosis of mental illness as clear in Lagos as it is in London. Information and research can be applied widely if a classification system is used, and it is clear that we are discussing the same illness. The classification system aims to be practical and versatile. Each mental illness is given a code, which you may have seen used on insurance claims forms as a form of shorthand.

The DSM4 is the *Fourth Diagnostic and Statistical Manual for Mental Disorders*, which was evolved by the Americans. It is the second important diagnostic manual that we have in use.

Both classifications are widely used and respected, and they complement each other.

Symptoms of depressive illness

These are some of the symptoms you may have had:

- *Sleep disturbance.* Classically someone wakes up at 3–4 am with their mind working overtime. 'It's as if I've got some unfinished business.' It is difficult to get back to sleep.
- *Sleep quality is poor.* Whether broken or heavy, people wake in the morning unrefreshed.
- *Appetite change.* Usually this is loss of appetite, but can appear as overeating.
- *Loss of sex drive.*
- *Constipation.*
- *Weight changes.* This could be weight gain or loss.
- *Lethargy,* or *restlessness* and *agitation.*

How depression affects how you feel

- Mood low, loss of pleasure, loss of interest in usual activities.
- Mood may vary through the day, tending to be worse in the mornings.
- Tears over little things.
- Poor self-esteem and self-image.
- Poor concentration (people can perform unexpectedly poorly at work).
- Indecisiveness, dithering.
- Feeling awfully guilty, or hostile and angry.
- Feeling useless and helpless.
- Lack of drive.
- Irritability and behaviour out of character.
- Disengaging, withdrawing from life.

Insomnia

I get insomnia, but my doctor won't give me sleeping pills; she seems to think I'm depressed but there's no earthly reason why I should be.

You don't have to have a reason to become depressed. Sometimes there is an obvious stress or life-event, but sometimes it just seems to overtake someone for no reason. Insight can be subtly affected so that you are the last person to realise how low you have become. It is understandable to feel that having depression means that you have failed in some way, that somehow you haven't made the grade, and that it's your fault. Once you have managed to get past these thoughts, you can get on with dealing with it – and making it better. Depression is an illness not a failing.

Insomnia means difficulty with sleeping. Difficulty getting off to sleep is usually a sign of stress and worry. If you are persistently waking up very early in the morning, perhaps at 4 am, that sort of sleep disturbance is likely to be associated with depression. It is important to make the connection because the right medication will then help.

Like your GP, most doctors are rather reluctant to give out sleeping tablets in this sort of situation for two reasons: first it is often best to try self-help methods, and secondly it may well be that a course of antidepressants (rather than sleeping pills) would be much more helpful in getting your sleep pattern re-established.

A few nights of good sleep makes a lot of difference to how we function; severe sleep deprivation is torture.

Why can't I get to sleep?

There are two patterns of sleep disturbance. If you are anxious and unsettled, worried about things happening in your life, then you may not get off to sleep easily. This is a common sign of anxiety and stress. A warm milky drink, a breath of fresh air, a quiet evening without too much excitement on the TV, a comfortable bed, will all help you settle down and get off to sleep naturally. Sleep is a habit and some people sleep more than others. It is said that we need less as we get older. Shift workers and aircrew have to put up with disturbed sleep patterns and may need an occasional sleeping tablet to correct their sleep pattern.

If you get off to sleep without difficulties, but then wake in the early hours, perhaps at 3–4 am, that is much more suggestive of depression. Persistent early morning wakening is one of the cast-iron signs of a depressive illness. It is caused by a shift in the body's chemistry as a result of the illness, and is often associated with anxiety and, particularly, low mood on awakening.

Some people sleep more than usual when depressed. They may feel tired all the time, and awake unrefreshed after a night's sleep.

Loss of drive

I'm a marathon runner, and I developed depression a few years ago. One of the first ways it affected me was that I lost the drive to train, it became harder and harder to keep fit and I couldn't understand why. Is this common?

It's not common, but this is certainly one of the 'atypical' ways in which depression can manifest itself. Competitive athletes have to focus on their fitness to the exclusion of much else on a daily basis, and they may have to overlook many of their own feelings to keep in training at a high level. Athletes in serious training, who get an injury or who have to reduce their activity for some other reason, do miss their exercise dreadfully. They are probably missing their own 'endorphins', nervous system chemicals produced during exercise. These naturally occurring opiates make you feel well; you can get feelings of withdrawal from them when you stop exercise, as well as feeling flatter in mood.

When athletic patients cannot train for some reason, they may be helped by burning up the same amount of energy in other ways; so runners with foot injuries may use the pool or the gym instead to keep fit, thus avoiding loss of their natural endorphins. You don't have to be a marathon runner, but taking up some exercise can be a really good way of improving your mood. Get off that sofa!

Loss of drive is often one of the subtler signs of depression. Those of us who are not athletes might experience it as a general lack of energy, and difficulty in getting started on anything, whether work projects or doing the laundry. Sex drive is often affected, and perhaps writer's block can be a form of this too.

Loss of weight

My aunt feels generally unwell and has lost weight. I was worried it might be cancer because my mum (her sister) had that, but she's had all sorts of scans and tests and they can't find anything wrong. Now they want to put her on antidepressants, even though she doesn't really feel depressed. Is this the right thing to do?

'Medically unexplained symptoms' are surprisingly common among people coming to see their family doctor. People often complain of dizziness, tiredness, headaches, poor sleep, chronic aches and pains in chest, back or abdomen. Research has shown that in only 10–15% of people with these symptoms is there any physical cause to be found. In the remainder, physical, social and psychological factors are probably combining in some complex way to produce the feeling that someone is ill.

For example, unrecognised tensions at work or in the family may cause someone unconsciously to clench their muscles. This muscle tension may cause headaches, back strains, or unexplained exhaustion; it's as if someone has had to run 5 miles even though they've been only sitting at their desk.

Our *autonomic nervous system* runs automatic bodily functions, such as blood pressure, breathing and heart rate, pain responses and gut activity. When this system responds to stress we may experience palpitations, or stomach aches and cramps ('irritable bowel syndrome'). Some people may breath faster when under stress, without realising it. This 'hyperventilation' causes dizziness, giddiness and, perhaps, unexplained tingling and numbness, especially in fingers and toes: this tingling also affects the area around your mouth. Overbreathing causes us to 'wash out' carbon dioxide from our bodies; this causes a subtle and temporary change in the acidity of the blood. This in turn causes the tingling by effecting a transient lowering of the chemical calcium in our blood.

Sometimes we are the last people to recognise our own pressures and stresses; yet they may be so obvious to a bystander.

Explaining why someone feels inexplicably ill is not always easy. Some people may clearly be worried about a particular major illness, such as cancer or AIDS, and once that is out in the open, and we both realise that is what they are worried about, we can start to deal with their concerns with appropriate tests. In other cases we may have to carry out extensive investigations to exclude any other illness. We have to be careful that these do not add to someone's anxiety about themselves, as the stress of waiting for investigations and results is, in itself, considerable. A referral to a specialist for a consultant overview can be most helpful in reassuring people that everything has been done, although it is also important not to chase around the Health Service for cures for the inexplicable.

What can be done to help her? She still feels awful, even though all the tests are normal. I don't think she's making it up.

Feeling awful is not imaginary. When a doctor comes across this type of problem, it is important that all medications are kept to a bare minimum, to reduce any chance of side-effects or odd drug reactions. Overinvestigation should be avoided – more and more X-rays, scans and other tests, unless new symptoms appear, will only add to further worry. We will look for sources of stress and strain, past or present, in people's lives. These symptoms do seem commoner in those who have had an unhappy childhood. Doctors look for obvious signs of depressive illness. A good night's sleep can make all the difference to one's well-being, and poor sleep can insidiously lower mood. Continuing worry about illness lowers mood too, as do continuing symptoms.

Finally, in large trials there is strong evidence of benefits from using antidepressant medication, whether or not people with these 'unexplained medical symptoms' were obviously depressed. Many people with this sort of picture are helped by long courses of low-dose antidepressants. There is also evidence that cognitive behavioural therapy (see Chapter 5), individually or in a group setting, is helpful.

Tiredness

I feel tired all the time. Is this likely to be a physical illness, or is it depression?

Fatigue is a very common complaint. At any one time about 20% of men and about 30% of women will say that they feel tired all the time.

The majority of younger women in the UK have a job and a family, and the working day is long. Sleep may be disrupted by young children. Efforts to remain physically fit may be thwarted because of time constraints.

The situation is no less difficult for most working men. Stresses of work, plus taking much more responsibility for child care and running the house, often make the 'new man' a stressed and tired man.

If the tiredness is sufficiently troublesome to warrant seeing the doctor, the commonest reason for feeling 'tired all the time' is mild depression and anxiety. Antidepressants may be of help in this situation. Other common causes are continuing stress and difficulties.

There are also some common and easily treatable physical causes for tiredness, which include iron deficiency anaemia (common in women of child-bearing age), thyroid gland disorders and, occasionally, the bowel disorder, coeliac disease, which might cause few signs except fatigue. The physical causes are much less common that the 'social' causes.

What causes it? What can I do about it?

Stress, worry, and anxiety can all cause exhaustion. Having your muscles unconsciously tense from stress and strain leaves you feeling as though you've run a marathon at the end of the day – even if you've not been out of doors. Doing too much is obviously tiring, but more insidious is the sort of tiredness people get when they become out of condition, get run down, and stop taking any exercise. Little things like an uncomfortable bed, a noisy bedroom, too many late nights can all contribute. You can get too tired to relax.

Some people may have a particular worry, and getting this out into the open can be a great relief. Others need to make some life change to improve how they feel: a job that's not right for you, a relationship that you're not happy in, housing that isn't satisfactory.

We all know that holidays are good for you. If you can't take a break soon, try to wind down and reduce all your responsibilities for a couple of weeks. Then start an exercise programme, to get back into condition. Gradually build up your level of physical

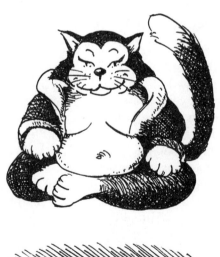

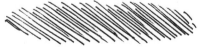

activity; you don't have to run marathons, but aim to make yourself feel out of breath for 20 minutes, 3 times weekly.

Look after yourself: good nutrition, healthy sleep, and social recreation are important. Make sure that you have something enjoyable to look forward to in your week. Relaxation techniques such as yoga, breathing exercises or meditation will all help keep tension – and hence tiredness – under control.

Diagnosis of depressive illness

Depressive illness cannot be diagnosed by a blood test or a scan – there is no single test that can diagnose depression with certainty. What the doctor is looking for is evidence that a person is ill, and ill with depression – they are not able to function normally and they feel different. They feel that they have changed, and are 'not themselves'. The doctor will ask questions about your symptoms. The person who is depressed will experience many of the changes described.

What's the point of seeing a doctor about my moods anyway? Surely they're my own business?

We all have differing moods, they are our own business, and they're all part of what we like to call life's rich tapestry. The world would be a very bland place if everyone was in the same mood all the time. Moods are our natural reaction to what happens in our lives. Sadness follows a loss, anxiety follows a threat, and these moods help us deal with life; but sometimes a bad mood is prolonged and does not naturally return to a comfortable level. Persistent disturbances of mood can cause poor functioning and loss of ability. When your moods interfere with your enjoyment of life, illness might be developing.

Depressive illness is a curious condition. Unlike most other illnesses, quite often someone who has become persistently low and sad is the last to recognise that they have changed. Sometimes there is a very obvious reason why someone is upset;

sometimes our moods change without obvious causes, perhaps for quite deep-seated reasons. Physical illness can trigger off depression, so can certain drugs (official and otherwise). Even the climate can perhaps affect some people.

When your level of functioning is affected – for longer than a couple of weeks – it's sensible to consider seeking help.

My wife's had lots of tests in hospital for suspected stomach ulcers. Nothing has shown up but she still feels awful and has lost weight. The doctors are saying it's depression. How could this make her feel so ill?

Maybe a third of people who are investigated for common symptoms such as stomach disorders, or chest pain have no abnormality that can be found. All the tests, such as endoscopy (looking inside the stomach with a video camera), blood tests and barium X-ray come out normal. We know that a depressive illness can underlie these symptoms.

Perhaps the best analogy is of the molehill being turned into a mountain by depression, which subtly affects the many ways we perceive how our own bodies are working. Most people get some sort of indigestion at times, but, if you are run down and depressed, the fairly minor aches and pains from this can be magnified. If you have some worries, or feel that it just might be cancer, you are less likely to be reassured by normal test results. Having these tests done can in itself be quite stressful and make you more anxious.

In this situation it is often helpful to let some time pass, and to keep in touch for review. Then we can look at any new symptoms and reconsider the question of depression once they have had a chance to digest what we've said. It is important for doctor and patient to keep an open mind.

What does the term 'dual-diagnosis' mean?

Dual-diagnosis is a term that is used when someone has a combination of a psychiatric illness plus a problem with alcohol or substance abuse. Some people may be more vulnerable to substance abuse because of their depression or other psychiatric conditions; others may be trying to control their own feelings by 'medicating' themselves with alcohol or street drugs. Perhaps a third of substance abusers have an underlying psychiatric condition. This may be masked by their drug or alcohol use, and presents a double challenge to medical care.

Until both conditions are recognised as being present, it will be hard to make much progress. Expert psychiatric assessment is generally needed to unravel this sort of situation. Unrecognised, the second problem will interfere with treatment of the first one.

Where can I get help?

Start with your General Practitioner. A physical check-up, and some blood tests may be helpful to exclude any medical condition that could be making you run down. Talking always helps, so try to confide in a friend or family member. The Samaritans or the Saneline hotline (see Appendix 1), local clergy, school or work counsellors, NHS Direct or your local NHS Walk-in Centre can also help you to take the first step.

Don't put up with it, do something about it. Part of being depressed is feeling that nothing can or will help. That's untrue. Depressive illness is eminently treatable.

Why is a brain scan recommended for some depressed people?

Brain scans are of two main types: CAT (computed axial tomography) and MRI (magnetic resonance imaging). The MRI scan tends to give a much more detailed picture of the anatomy of your brain. Very rarely the development of a resistant, or atypical depressive illness, is associated with the presence of a brain lesion (an area of damage of some sort). Sometimes, a small stroke is the unrecognised cause or, very rarely indeed, a brain tumour (most often benign). Brain scans can pick up, or more usually exclude, such lesions. The first onset of depression in late life may be associated with dementia (such as Alzheimer's disease), and a brain scan may be able to demonstrate some atrophy (brain wasting) in these circumstances. Other types of brain scan (PET, SPECT) are at present of research interest, but not of clinical usefulness, in depression.

My GP has referred me to a psychiatrist. Does that mean I'm going mad?

No. It does mean that you are going to have a longer and more detailed assessment, and a specialist opinion on the best treatment for you. Most – perhaps 90% – cases of depression are managed well by GPs. The more complicated cases, for example where there hasn't been a good response to treatment, are referred for a consultant opinion, and this can also give you access to more treatment resources, such as hospital-based therapies.

2
Who gets depressive illness?

Anyone can get this illness: we are all potentially at risk. People of all ages, from every culture and every socioeconomic group can become ill with depression. What differs in different ages and cultures may be the way that the illness shows itself.

Depressive illness in a teenager may look very different from depressive illness in an old person. The depressed teenager may be very tired, lacking in energy and irritable. The depressed older person may be restless, tense and sleepless. Depressive illness in, for example, rural India may show itself with extreme concern and distress about physical complaints rather than tearfulness and low mood, which may be the dominant features seen in a depressed European. The illness, whoever it affects and whenever it strikes, is equally disabling but differently expressed.

In this chapter we discuss some specific groups of people who may become depressed, and the different ways in which they may be affected, including children, adolescents, women who have recently had babies or have reached the menopause (and discuss whether men may experience anything similar), older people, people addicted to alcohol and drugs, people with seasonal affective disorder (SAD) or chronic fatigue syndrome. We also talk about how bereavement, shock and injury or violence can trigger off a depressive illness.

Depression in children

Depressive symptoms or features (as opposed to depressive illness) are common in emotionally disturbed children. Serious depressive illness in children is very uncommon and may occur in about 1 in 1000 children aged 10–11. Less severe depression occurs in about 2 children in 100. Much more commonly in children, depression is expressed as a behavioural disorder, or shows itself with bodily complaints, e.g. worry about health, abdominal pain, headache and fatigue. Deliberate self-harm and suicide are exceedingly rare before adolescence. Teenagers' worries about growing up often include weight, appearance, relationships, sexual orientation, and what other people will think about them. All of these difficulties are helped by talking, although some – such as being uncertain about one's sexual orientation – may still not be easy to discuss nowadays.

Children and adolescents can be treated with antidepressants. Usually the newer antidepressant drugs (SSRIs) seem to be more effective than the old-fashioned drugs. A central and key part of treating a child or adolescent who is depressed is working with the family to help them make necessary changes. Involving school or college is not only advisable but is likely to be extremely helpful in the treatment of a depressed young person. Depression in a child or adolescent may be a sign that something very serious is wrong in the family, the environment or at school. Looking at, and trying to deal, with difficult social, family or school situations may do as much as, if not more than, medication can usually do.

Adolescence and depression

Before puberty the rates of depression in boys and girls are equal. After puberty twice as many girls as boys become depressed.

About 5 adolescents in 100 become depressed. Depressive illness in adolescents can be difficult to spot. Anger, irritability, withdrawing from friends and alienation from parents, academic underachieving, low self-esteem and sadness may all indicate depression – or be a reflection of the challenges and turmoil of normal adolescence. The changes brought about by depressive illness in adults are also seen in adolescents, but sleep disturbance is less common (adolescents are famously good at sleeping!). Delusions (abnormal beliefs) and hallucinations (abnormal perceptions) are less common than in adults.

Depression in adolescents, as in adults, may be linked to excess alcohol. Parents are often unaware of how much their child drinks – the average alcohol intake in a 15-year-old is 7 units a week. Some will drink nothing, others the average amount, and others far more. Adolescents may start to drink to try and make themselves feel better. The same is true of street drugs. Once alcohol or substances are used regularly, secondary problems occur. Finding the money to fund the habit becomes very difficult, and the problems rapidly compound. There is more information about alcohol and substance abuse later in this chapter.

The disturbing rise in suicide rates in 15 to 19-year-olds may well be linked to the increase in alcohol consumption and the use of street drugs in this age group. It is never helpful to think that your child would 'never do such a thing'. There is huge peer pressure on adolescents to drink or take street drugs – they are all very vulnerable.

My daughter is 14 and I think she's really depressed. I know how she feels because I went through the same thing in my late teens. I've asked my GP about putting her on Prozac or something similar, but she seems reluctant. Shouldn't she prescribe it for her?

Teenagers and younger children can certainly become seriously depressed. Adolescents need careful treatment because they are going through all the stresses of adolescence, because they are growing rapidly and facing all sorts of new challenges in their lives, and not least because it's not easy to know what they're thinking. Also, children might go to the doctor with physical symptoms, so that depression is visually very hard to recognise. Antidepressants of some sort may well be very helpful for your daughter.

However, many GPs would wish to ask the advice of a psychiatrist with special skills in this situation rather than engage in treatment of someone so young themselves. There are specialised counselling services for teenagers such as Off the Record (see Appendix 1) but, if she seems seriously depressed at her age, she definitely needs medical attention too. Ask the doctor to refer her to a child psychiatrist.

My nephew was treated for depression aged 18. He's OK now, and at University, but takes his final exams next year. We're worried how he'll cope with the stress.

First of all, make sure he knows that you are helpfully concerned, that he can talk to you if he runs into a problem, and that you will keep in touch with him yourselves just as general friendly support. Looking after himself generally is important, and we have suggested a number of self-help tactics in Chapter 4.

Secondly, be sure that he is aware of the sources of help if he does start to feel under stress or overwhelmed. These start with his tutors, and would include the University Health Service, local counselling services (most Universities have their own counsellors) and phone help lines such as the Samaritans or a local Night Line service (see Appendix 1).

My teenage nephew used to be quiet and generally kept a low profile. Over the past few months he has taken to riding his motorbike very fast and has had a whole string of girlfriends.

The distinction between reckless behaviour and what normal young men do for fun may be a very fine line. There may be nothing wrong. Recklessness, however, can be part of a breakdown of normal behaviour in the setting of drinking too much, or taking street drugs – both of which numb judgement. The risk-taking behaviour can also include unprotected sexual activity or having sex with multiple partners. Any marked change in behaviour in a young man should alert those around him to the possibility of substance misuse. Occasionally some more risky behaviour emerges from self-destructive thoughts arising in a depressive illness.

Women

Postnatal problems

My wife became very withdrawn and low when she had our last baby, and the doctor said it was postnatal depression – how should it be treated?

After having a baby, about 50% of women experience postnatal blues with fleeting low mood and tearfulness lasting for 1–2 days. It most often occurs on day 3. Though it can be uncomfortable, it is brief and gets better spontaneously.

More serious is postnatal depression, which can occur in about 1 in 10 women, most frequently in the first month after delivery. Postnatal depression lasts longer and can without treatment go on for several months. It is more likely in older mothers, those who were separated from their father when they were young, where there were physical problems in the pregnancy and around the birth of the baby, and in those having a past history of depression. Most postnatal depressive illnesses last for less than a month (even without treatment). If it lingers, it is important to get it treated promptly.

The treatment is as for any other depressive illness, with the proviso that, if your wife wants to breastfeed the baby, the drugs are chosen with special care. The drugs that we have most experience with during breastfeeding are the long-established tricyclic antidepressants like doxepin (Sinequan). Fluoxetine (Prozac), a newer antidepressant, has also been very widely used. It is, of course, very important not just to be prescribed drugs but to have plenty of 'talking time', and as much help available for her and the baby as possible. Postnatal depression is likely to be difficult for you as well. Sometimes it is very helpful to have a limited amount of therapy and guidance as a couple. See Chapter 5 for more information on treatment.

Can postnatal depression recur after another pregnancy?

Yes. There is an increased risk of depression following subsequent pregnancies (about twice the average risk), but it is by no means inevitable. It is important to remember that having been depressed in the past will almost certainly mean that the mother will realise what is happening much faster than during the first illness – as will family members. The GP and health visitor will also be alert for any changes of early depression, and treatment can be started quickly.

Menopause

Does the menopause cause depression?

No. There is a widely held folk belief that it does, but careful review of research shows that the menopause itself does not cause depression. However, around the time of the menopause (average age 51) there are several very big life changes and adjustments that may be happening. This is the time when children are leaving home. Remaining children are often (potentially) difficult teenagers. Parents, and in-laws, may be ill and need care or may die. Husbands may be ill for the first time. There may be the threat of redundancy. Growing old is, perhaps for the first time, a tangible reality. The fifth decade is a time when both men and women tend to review and reflect about what they have done with their lives. It can sometimes be a time of regret. It is these sorts of changes and losses that can lead to depression rather than the actual fact of the menopause.

Can HRT help depression that occurs around the time of the menopause?

Yes it can. HRT will not act as an antidepressant, however, but can be expected to help decrease some of the unpleasant symptoms that can occur during the menopause, such as hot flushes and night sweats. Sleep is sometimes seriously disrupted with night sweating, and this will tend to make coping with low mood much more difficult. Sleep that has been disrupted by menopausal symptoms can continue to be disrupted even when the changes of the menopause are settled – a pattern of poor sleep can be established. It is important to try and treat this early.

Victims of violence

My sister says that her husband is violent towards her. I can't understand why she stays with him.

Domestic violence accounts for about a quarter of violent crime within the UK, but only about a third of incidents are reported. Domestic violence is the leading cause of injury in women aged 20–44 years. The rate of violence is the same in all the social classes. About two women a week are killed by their partners in the UK. It is a very serious problem. Violence tends to escalate, and worsen, as long as the victim stays with their aggressive partner. Sadly domestic violence does not get better with time. Women are most at risk of being victims of domestic violence when they are pregnant.

There are many reasons – not least practical ones – for staying with a violent partner. It may be very difficult to get away from the home; there may be no spare money for taxis or train fares. It can be extremely difficult to find accommodation at very short notice for a mother and perhaps two or three children. There is always a very real fear of reprisals for the woman who escapes.

Victims of domestic violence tend to become 'dis-empowered'. A situation develops which is very like that which exists between a prisoner and a jailer. The victim is undermined and gradually loses the necessary energy and self-esteem to stand back from the situation and see what is really happening. Violent men are often very vulnerable and may come from abusive backgrounds. Their vulnerability can produce a feeling of pity and caring from the victim. There is a belief on her part that she can change him if she tries hard enough. Violent men can of course change, but they often need considerable help and support to do so. It is too dangerous a problem to try and address alone.

What could my sister do?

She could encourage her husband to seek help. Groups such as 'Men Against Violence' (see Appendix 1) may be a good starting point. Domestic violence is often linked to alcohol abuse. This will need to be addressed. The perpetrator could be encouraged to contact AA, and the family can gain considerable help and support by contacting Al-Anon (see Appendix 1).

It is not helpful to keep the problem secret. Reporting domestic violence to the police may well be the first step in tackling and dealing with the problem. The police have made great efforts to change the way they deal with victims of domestic violence. Women are now treated much more sympathetically when they report domestic violence than even just a few years ago.

If violence is continuing and the perpetrator seems unable or unwilling to accept responsibility for what is happening, it is essential that any victim of domestic violence has an emergency plan in place, which would enable her to leave the home at very short notice. This may include keeping some spare cash ('getaway money') aside, keeping a second set of car keys available, having access to a friend or relative for shelter, and having the telephone number of Social Services readily available. The Social Services Department can provide a 'safe-house' for battered women and their children in an emergency. The addresses of safe-houses are kept confidential, and change, for obvious reasons.

Finally for a victim of violence, having somebody who will listen, and encourage them to try and alter the situation and seek help, will be of enormous importance. Being angry and condemning the violence does not help either the victim or the perpetrator of violence to work for change.

I wake up at night with horrible dreams and am very irritable since I was mugged. What help can I get?

Any violent experience to ourselves is very shocking. It's as if the safety of our personal space has been invaded. Broken sleep, recurrent thoughts about the assault, mood changes and irritability are all a normal psychological reaction in these circumstances. Victims may irrationally blame themselves after an assault ('If I hadn't said that, he wouldn't have done it') and self-esteem is lost. There is shock and humiliation at our lost safety or self-respect.

These understandable feelings can pass on their own with time but it does seem that specialised counselling helps. The Victim Support Scheme (VSS) (see Appendix 1) is a highly recommended national charity with branches in many areas. Their brief is to support anyone injured as the result of a criminal act. They work free with trained volunteer counsellors who can visit people at home. They can also assist in workplaces with staff support schemes.

Men

Do men get the menopause too? My husband is not quite himself now he's nearly 50. He keeps mentioning his age and says he looks old.

Men may not visit the doctor with classical symptoms of depression and therefore it may go undiagnosed for some time. The 'male menopause' is something you'll see discussed more in newspaper articles than in medical journals. Men do not undergo the same dramatic step down in hormonal function that women do, but they do go through the same life changes in middle age as women do. Children become independent and leave home, leaving the domestic nest empty. Younger people at work may be coming up fast on the inside lane, maybe making them feel that they have got as far as they can in their careers. Their life roles might be changing in subtle ways, and they realise that they are not indispensable. They may start to experience ill-health (minor or major) in middle age for the first time. None of these factors in themselves is overwhelming, but all can contribute to a perhaps subtle drop in self-esteem and loss of vitality. There is ongoing research into male hormones, and how they affect mood. It is an exciting new area.

What can I do about it?

One way of looking at this is to consider that he has the choice of using his interests and skills for 'recreation' or of just stagnating. Encouraging him to develop new interests and hobbies can be a great help. Perhaps at your age the children will be leaving home, and for the first time for some years he will find that he has time on his hands. Spending time together on interests that you used to share, things that you had in common when you first settled down together, is a good start.

Elderly

My granny is 89, and has been in hospital for months since breaking her leg. She seems very quiet and low, not her usual self at all, and hasn't got back on her legs yet. What can be done?

Depression can affect up to a quarter of hospital medical patients. The probable causes are many: the upsets in their daily routine, pain, loss of social contacts, and the effects of complicated medication. This isn't always easy to spot, as they tend to be very uncomplaining, and the doctors and nurses might not notice that someone has lost their spark.

This can sometimes explain why an older person is slow to recover after an operation, or slow to get moving after a fracture. Start off by discussing this with the Ward Sister or Doctor. Elderly people can respond brilliantly to medication for depression.

Isn't sleeping poorly and feeling low just part of getting old?

Depressive illness in older people is common and easily overlooked by family and doctors. About a quarter of over 65-year-old people seeing their family doctor will have depression. Maybe 1 in 3 people living in residential homes are depressed. The illness can be missed because the distress is expressed in bodily complaints, rather than the experience of low mood.

Reduced sleep, weight loss, poor appetite, constipation, mood swings and general slowing down can all be part of the subtle picture of depression in an older person, and many of these symptoms may wrongly be ascribed to growing old. Picking this condition up in older people is important because treatment can improve the quality of life immensely.

Bereavement

Our grandad has been very low, since he was widowed. He keeps talking about moving to the seaside where he grew up, but that was 50 years ago and he won't know anybody there. We don't think this is sensible.

Nor would we, but it is not uncommon for elderly depressed people to make unrealistic or romantic plans, for example to return to their home town to look up old friends. They can disregard the obvious practical difficulties (including their own infirmities) and are somehow hoping to turn the clock back to a golden past – which perhaps never existed. Major life decisions such as selling up and moving house must be discouraged when someone is bereaved. If possible, delay decisions about major changes for at least a year after bereavement, possibly even two. Try to steer round the subject – 'Until you are better, Grandad.'

My father is 76 and has become very quiet, withdrawn and forgetful since mum died. Sometimes I find him in tears. Is he getting senile? What can be done?

Depressive illness in the elderly can be difficult to spot. A depressed elderly person can appear to have a dementing illness. If the depression is treated, the 'dementia' fades. On the other hand, dementia can first show itself with low mood.

Finally, your father's poorer functioning could be a result of his grieving process. Bereavement can be all-consuming and, at times, difficult to distinguish from a depressive illness.

Your father needs a review by his doctor. It would be very helpful if you could attend too, in order to explain the changes you have seen. Once it is clear what is causing this, he can then start treatment.

Post-traumatic stress disorder

After a bad road traffic accident, I am physically fine, but am depressed and very tense. Is this PTSD?

It may be. Post-traumatic stress disorder (PTSD) can occur when somebody is exposed to a traumatic event outside the normal range of human experience. That experience would cause suffering in almost everybody. The response that occurs includes intense fear and a feeling of helplessness. This can lead on to persistent 'replays' or flashbacks of the incident with recurrent nightmares, very intense psychological distress and the physical symptoms of extreme anxiety, when the person is exposed to any situation that might resemble or remind the person of the trauma.

Because these flashbacks are so unpleasant, the person often goes to great lengths to avoid any of the situations that cause them. People with PTSD are described as being 'hyper-aroused'. They are in a state of high anxiety and alertness. They easily become startled, their sleep is disturbed and they tend to be hyper- or overvigilant about their surroundings. These symptoms cause a decrease in the person's general ability to cope. Depression commonly occurs as a consequence of the PTSD.

Can it be treated?

Yes. PTSD responds to a variety of treatments. It usually responds best to cognitive behaviour therapy (see Chapter 5). The person is encouraged to relive the experience in a graded and safe way, while at the same time taught techniques to relax. Learning more about a process of the illness and the way in which stress affects the body can make unexplained and frightening symptoms much more manageable. People suffering with PTSD quite frequently become depressed and this will need treating, perhaps with medication, in its own right. Some anti-depressants are prescribed in PTSD, not necessarily to treat depression, but to control symptoms of anxiety. Antidepressants have the added advantage that they are not addictive, whereas some medications that control anxiety very well (like Valium and its family) are addictive and cannot be used for long periods.

Sometimes people suffering from PTSD try to blot out their anxiety by using alcohol. This tends to compound the problem since, after initial relaxation with alcohol, there will be a rebound of very unpleasant anxiety, which will make the situation worse. (See also Chapter 5 on Treatment and Chapter 8 on Benefits.)

Other medical disorders

Seasonal affective disorder (SAD)

Someone told me about a condition called SAD. How does this affect you?

SAD stands for seasonal affective disorder – mood disorder related to the seasons of the year. Some people do describe feeling particularly low during the dark winter months. Of course, good weather cheers everybody up, and bad weather can make one gloomy, but for a few people seasonal climate changes do appear to trigger off real symptoms of depression. It seems to relate to shorter daylight hours. It seems that these people are particularly sensitive to the stimulating effects of sunlight.

How common is it?

One study of 443 Aberdeen nurses found that 3% had SAD, and about 10% had a milder form of SAD. Twice as many women suffer from it as men, and it seems to start in people in their 30s.

How is it different from ordinary depression?

People still get typical depressive symptoms of feeling low, irritable and having a lack of energy. However, rather than loss of appetite and weight, and early morning waking, people with SAD may sleep more heavily than usual, eat more and put on weight – almost as if they're going into hibernation – and of course they describe a clearcut seasonal variation.

How can I tell if I've got it?

The term is applied if you have had 3 or more episodes of mood disorder within the same 90-day period of the year, for 3 or more consecutive years. There will also be a pattern of improvement, and remission, within another 90-day period of the year.

These are the strict research criteria for the illness. However, many people who have a tendency to be depressed might show their own particular pattern of relapse. The winter and early spring are often difficult, but some can become ill in the summer or autumn. Other factors then come into play – it may be the anniversary of a bereavement, or the breakdown of a marriage, for instance.

Chronic fatigue syndrome

I think I've got ME. My doctor says it doesn't exist and that I have chronic fatigue. What is the difference?

ME is an abbreviation for myalgic encephalomyelitis. This is not a widely accepted term, since there is no real scientific evidence that there is an isolated illness process involving muscles and the brain that accounts for the symptoms of fatigue. The great difficulty with using the label ME is that there is an expectation that rest, and more rest, is the treatment of choice. This has been challenged. What is perhaps more helpful, is to say that there are a significant number of people who become chronically fatigued – or tired all the time. In some people this follows a clearly defined viral infection. Their fatigue can be incapacitating and very debilitating. Because there are no diagnostic tests for chronic fatigue, it does not mean that it is imaginary. It is a very real illness with very real and serious consequences. There do seem to be links with stress.

If you had the viral illness and were stressed at that time, you are more likely to have developed postviral fatigue, than someone who was not stressed. Also, there is an increased risk of chronic fatigue developing if there was an uncertainty about what caused the original illness. People who can be given a clear diagnosis from the outset of their viral illness are much less likely to develop chronic fatigue.

Can chronic fatigue be treated?

Very definitely it can. One of the main problems, however, is that, if you feel very weak and vulnerable, you may not feel able to cooperate with the treatment. The fatigue will need to be consistently and gently challenged.

Treatment will include a system of graded exercise (gradually increasing physical activity). There should be a new routine about times to get up in the mornings and to go to bed at night, and a schedule for taking naps. It is often helpful to keep a diary of activity achieved, and feelings. This might well show a connection between daily stress and levels of fatigue.

Finally, if mood is low (and it often is), or there is excessive anxiety present, it could be very helpful to take an antidepressant (see Chapter 5) Any medication taken is normally started at a very low dose and increased slowly depending on progress. People with chronic fatigue are perhaps more likely to experience side-effects from medication – hence the slow start.

This package of treatment can be reasonably expected to produce significant improvement in at least two-thirds of sufferers. Treatments advocating very long periods of rest and special diets are very unlikely to produce good results and may indeed be positively harmful.

Can dental fillings or diet cause chronic fatigue?

No. There is no good evidence that dental fillings, or diet (particularly yeast in the diet), cause fatigue. There is also no good evidence that candida (a yeast infection) causes chronic fatigue, although this is often suggested by alternative therapy practitioners.

People who have chronic fatigue are often desperate for help and very vulnerable. They will 'try anything' in an attempt to feel better. Generally speaking, *the more extreme the treatment* (and sometimes the more expensive) *the less it is likely to help.*

Dementia

**Grandad is 69, and he's becoming increasingly forgetful
and slow. He left the gas on the other day and got lost
when he went shopping. He doesn't seem his usual self at
all. Would antidepressants help him?**

Probably not. Failing memory in the elderly, together with
reduced functioning – such as poor personal hygiene or loss of
social ability – is more likely to indicate the onset of dementia.
The commonest causes are poor circulation within the brain
(causing mini-strokes), or Alzheimer's disease, a condition which
damages brain tissue itself. It is not part of normal ageing,
although it is normal for older people's memories to gently
become weaker as time goes by; 10% of over 65-year-olds, and
20% of over 80-year-olds have this illness.

Relatives are often the first to recognise that someone is
suffering from dementia. The following features can all become
evident as part of this condition:

- increased forgetfulness
- poor judgement
- coarsening of the personality
- irritability
- loss of interest in usual hobbies and social activities
- getting in a muddle when away from usual routine
- not recognising people
- difficulty in expressing oneself.

People may have little insight, and not realise that they are
becoming less able in this way.

When a person – or more likely a relative – comes with these
concerns, a physical examination is needed to exclude any
treatable reason why they may not be functioning well. Thyroid
disease, severe anaemia, kidney failure, vitamin deficiency,
tumours, certain infectious diseases, or the side-effects of other
medication are among the possible causes of deteriorating mental
functioning in older people that we can do something about.
Severe depression can also present in this way.

People with dementia place great pressures on their carers. Sadly, these conditions are likely to be progressive, and it is important that carers receive support from both Health and Social Services. Home helps, day care, meals on wheels, laundry services, the Attendance Allowance and other benefits, can all help to support those living at home. People who are more severely ill may need residential placements. Support groups can be a great help to carers.

Alcoholism

There is a question about teenagers and alcohol earlier in this chapter.

Is depression part of recovery from alcoholism?

Abuse of alcohol and other substances, such as street drugs, is associated with depression, because of their effect on neuro-transmitter levels (see Chapter 3). It is not unusual for a temporary depression to occur during substance abuse or after withdrawal. It is sometimes difficult to say which came first: the depression or the drink, but these depressive episodes are often self-limited. If this sort of depression does not resolve within 4–6 weeks, antidepressant medication may well be necessary. Anyone who has been drinking heavily will have noticed adverse effects on their mood. Mood and well-being continue to improve for several months after abstinence.

Coming back into the real world can be very difficult for people who are overcoming alcohol or drug problems. They need to put new ways of coping with life's stresses into place. Organisations such as AA or NA provide group support (see Appendix 1), and maybe one-to-one help from other people who have 'been there and done that' themselves. This includes ways that others have found to get by, tactics and strategies for surviving. When your mood is low and brittle, small problems – an unexpectedly large electricity bill, or just a funny look from a colleague – can become quite large difficulties to overcome.

Of those who fail to stop drinking, many simply have not got coping mechanisms in place to deal with day-to-day problem. They fall back on their favourite remedy, the one that always works for a while – and relapse.

My dad gets very low and drinks a lot. He is also very depressed. Are the two things linked?

They could well be. A considerable number of people use alcohol to try and feel better when they are depressed. They can sometimes go on to develop an alcohol dependence problem. Alcohol will make a depressed person feel better fleetingly. However, alcohol is a mood-altering drug – for every period of relaxation, there will be some rebound anxiety. Secondly, alcohol is a very powerful depressor of mood. Alcohol misuse is a potent cause of depressive illness. People who are depressed should attempt to cut down their alcohol intake to very modest levels. This in itself may well help the mood considerably.

What can I do to help someone who gets low and drinks too much?

Try not to be judgmental. They are likely to be feeling very bad about what is happening. Point out the low mood may be there because of the drinking, so encourage them to cut down. People are often reluctant to admit that they are drinking too much. There is confidential advice available from AA or other helplines (see Appendix 1). Your GP would also be very willing to discuss this. Al-Anon is a very helpful organisation for relatives/loved ones or people who are abusing alcohol. They give clear guidance about how to help and, equally important, what not to do. There is a tendency to take over the responsibility from the person who is drinking, or 'facilitate' the drinking.

I can't get to sleep without a large drink. Does that really matter?

Yes it does. A *small* measure of alcohol can help you drop off to sleep, but if you have large drinks, you will disturb your sleep rhythm. You will sleep well initially (you are anaesthetised), but will wake later, then quite frequently. A restless night follows when the alcohol effect wears off.

Alcohol dampens down REM sleep (rapid eye movement sleep). This is much needed and, if curtailed, will result in unrefreshing sleep.

How much alcohol is too much?

The Health Minister suggests a weekly healthy limit of 14 units for women and 21 for men. This is because women metabolise alcohol less effectively and risk very serious physical consequences of alcoholism. Cirrhosis in women, for example, tends to occur after a lower overall intake of alcohol than in men.

A unit is half a pint of ordinary beer (not strong lager or what we Bristolians call Turbocider), or a pub measure of wine or a single shot of spirits. It's good advice to have alcohol-free days too. Enjoy alcohol as a treat not as a habit. Have it as a blessing, not as a curse. Never use alcohol as a drug.

Drug abuse

My grandson is 16 and has become very moody. I know he smokes cannabis. He just sits in his room all the time, and doesn't seem to want to go out with friends. Is smoking cannabis harmful to him? Isn't it addictive?

Teenagers do often go through the most awful moody phases. Another thing that teenagers tend to do is experiment with whatever they come across, particularly if it is likely to be the subject of parental disaproval. Although pretty hair-raising for parents, this is a natural part of growing up, and is an important part of the process of finding one's own limits. We poor old parents just have to try to indicate what's safe and what isn't, be reasonably consistent, perhaps under provocation that would try the patience of a saint, and 'be there for them'.

In the scale of awful things that teenagers can get up to, smoking cannabis is certainly less harmful than making yourself violently sick with too much vodka, certainly much less harmful than sniffing glue or taking stimulant drugs such as Ecstasy, and nowhere near as dangerous as playing around with the very addictive hard drugs such as heroin, which are now horribly cheap. However, despite the recent changes in its legal status, it can still get you into trouble or excluded from school. There is an argument that someone who sells you cannabis may also sell you something worse if you have the money.

Anything carried to excess can cause problems, and some people seem more vulnerable to getting into trouble with this sort of thing than others. Contrary to popular belief, cannabis can be addictive – some people do become very heavy cannabis smokers. They may demonstrate mild but definite features of addiction, such as tolerance, craving and withdrawal symptoms. Because cannabis has a very long half-life (that's the time it stays in the blood stream), withdrawal symptoms may occur over a period of weeks in a mild form (rather than severely over a few hours, as happens with people who become addicted to alcohol). Occasionally, cannabis can be associated with a psychotic illness. It is not a harmless drug, but a potent mind-altering substance.

Sometimes it becomes apparent that unhappy or depressed teenagers are medicating themselves with street drugs of one form or another. They may be using drink or drugs to blot out difficult moods, horrid thoughts or bad feelings. Someone who doesn't socialise much may indeed be quietly becoming depressed. Someone who seems to be using drink or drugs heavily and is becoming a recluse, losing touch with their friends and interests is potentially in a very serious situation. Drawing them out of their shells can be pretty difficult. Perhaps the best way to start is by showing that you recognise that there is something wrong, and you realise that they are unhappy, by talking to them about it. Grannies can be very good at this.

I'm 19 and I do think I get depressed sometimes. Loads of my friends take 'E'(Ecstasy) in the clubs. I feel much more cheerful and lively when I do. Why shouldn't I?

Many people do take Ecstasy and it's certainly often used in clubs as part of the dance culture, but there are casualties – both physical ones, because of its effects on the heart (remember Leah Betts and others?) and the brain.

It is a stimulant drug, and is related to amphetamines. Amphetamines were given to exhausted pilots in the last war to keep them awake while flying, and were also used as an appetite suppressant in the 1950s and 1960s. Known as 'Purple Hearts', amphetamines became widely used as street drugs because of their stimulant effects (see the film *Quadrophrenia* for a picture of their use).

They mimic the effects of adrenaline release. This is the chemical that is released in the body in response to stress: the 'fight or flight' response. This raises your pulse, breathing rate, blood pressure, alertness, and dilates your pupils, but the amphetamine family of drugs are stimulants, not – repeat not – antidepressants. It is possible to feel agitated and depressed at the same time – an unpleasant experience. This group of drugs can merely make you feel more agitated, not happier.

The other downside of this group of drugs is that they are physically addictive. They can also lead, when used heavily, to really unpleasant paranoid feelings, even to a psychotic breakdown, a loss of contact with reality. They are dangerous in the setting of normal mood too. The effects can be unpredictable and sometimes catastrophic. They are best totally avoided.

P.S. They're illegal too – getting arrested is really bad for you!

Schizophrenia

Can depression turn into schizophrenia? My daughter was very depressed as a teenager, then had a serious breakdown in her 20s. The psychiatrist says she has a form of schizophrenia.

Depression does not turn into schizophrenia. They are separate illnesses, but they can coexist. However, schizophrenia can sometimes announce itself with a depressive episode. There can be a general feeling of unease and change, educational performance can fall off, and mood become very low and apathetic. Some months later, a much clearer picture may emerge, with signs of a schizophrenic illness (see below).

The situation can be more complex again. Young adults can develop a schizoaffective disorder. This means an illness in which there are changes in mood (up, down, or mixed), plus some schizophrenic features – perhaps hearing voices, or feeling controlled. This illness is usually brisk in onset and there are clear stresses leading up to it – perhaps the breakdown of a relationship.

The schizoaffective disorder almost always has a clear beginning and end, and it does not linger. Once over the episode, the person can look back on the illness and see it for what it was.

My son's personality just seems to have changed. He's lost his job, doesn't bother with his friends, and neglects himself. He seems bothered, sluggish and depressed. He won't talk to us about it. Could he be suffering from depression?

He certainly needs a medical assessment to see what is the matter. Someone whose personality changes so greatly could be at the beginning of a psychotic illness. This is likely to be something more serious than just depression.

Schizophrenia is a psychotic illness involving loss of contact with reality. About 1% of the population suffer from it. Features include hallucinations, usually hearing voices and, rarely, seeing visions. People tend to lose their drive and interest in others, and become emotionally flat. Some may experience paranoid ideas, feeling that there is some conspiracy against them.

Schizophrenia is fairly evenly spread throughout the world: some areas, such as northern Sweden and the south-west of Ireland, have more people affected. There is now evidence that prompt treatment improves the outlook for people with schizophrenia. Early treatment with modern medication has transformed the lives of people with this long-term illness. Seeing a relative develop and try to cope with this sort of illness is a huge stress for a family. One mother said, 'It was a relief when at least we knew what it was.'

3

Causes of depression

We do not know exactly how depressive illness is caused, but we are learning more and more about it. There are many components: genetic vulnerability, stresses, 'life-events' – major milestones good *and* bad, and some physical illnesses. Once initiated, there are biochemical, psychological and sociological mechanisms that inflame, or perpetuate, the illness.

Genetics

The genetic influence in manic depressive illness is about twice as great as in unipolar depression (where the only mood change is depression). If you have a manic depressive illness, the chances of a close relative developing any mood illness are about 20%. If you have a unipolar depressive illness, the chances are about 10%.

Attempts have been made to separate out the influence of genes and environment. Are siblings affected by the same illness because they share genes, or because they have been brought up together? If you look at twins, this question can be partially answered. Monozygotic or identical twins are babies formed from one fertilised egg cell dividing into two individuals – they share the same genes. Dizygotic twins, on the other hand, grow in the womb together but are formed by two separate egg cells being fertilised. These individuals will not have the same genes.

If the twins are brought up together, you can assume their treatment is very similar. If they develop an illness with some genetic causation, you would, however, expect the identical twins to have higher rates of the illness than non-identical twins. This is the case in depression. For an identical twin whose twin develops manic depressive illness, there is a 70% risk that he or she will develop the illness too. In non-identical twins, the rate is much lower, at 20%.

The genetic effect shown in twin studies looking at unipolar depression in identical twins shows a rate of about 50% illness in the twin, and 25% in a non-identical twin.

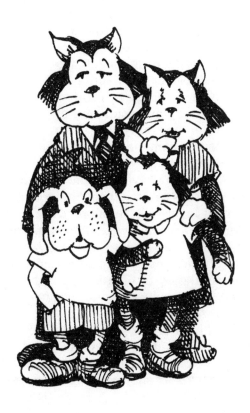

Neuro- (brain) chemistry theories of depression

Hippocrates in 400 BC established that everything we suffer comes from the brain – it always has been, and always will be, 'all in the mind'.

Mood and its disorders are closely linked with very basic brain functioning. People who are stressed show changes in their brain and body chemistry. Deep within the brain, the hypothalamus and the pituitary gland control the body's response to stress, either by increasing or decreasing their output of brain hormones. An increase in one of the hormones, CRF (corticotrophin-releasing factor), causes an outpouring of CRH (corticotrophin-releasing hormone). CRF-containing nerve cells are found throughout the brain.

If you put CRF into the brain of experimental animals, some of the symptoms of depression are mimicked – the animal stops eating adequately, its sleep rhythm changes, it stops grooming itself and it tends to neglect its offspring. This substance in turn, stimulates the pituitary gland to produce a chemical, which stimulates the adrenal glands (located above the kidneys) to make steroids, including cortisol. If stressed, we produce cortisol. The stresses can be of any kind – it could be a bereavement, a physical illness, or bullying. There is evidence now that depressed people have some increase in the size of the adrenal glands – stress is causing them to work extra hard. These changes in steroid levels are thought to affect the chemical transmitters – or neurotransmitters in the brain – and might, over a period of time, cause a depressive reaction to stress.

The probable physical explanation for depression is the so-called 'monoamine' theory of depression. If the brain becomes depleted of the monoamines, noradrenaline and serotonin, depression often results. Reserpine was a drug used in the treatment of high blood pressure. It was found to lower the levels of noradrenaline and serotonin in the brain (as well as lowering blood pressure), and it was noted that depression often followed. Research in the late 1960s showed levels of noradrenaline and serotonin in the brain were lower in depressed people than in normal people. Drugs that caused the opposite effect (that is, encouraged the level of neurotransmitters to rise) have the effect of elevating mood, if it was low before (not if it was already normal).

Neurotransmitters

This next section is rather technical, but there is no easy way to explain the chemical processes that are going on inside our brains. Our brains function by a series of chemicals being exchanged, which causes different messages producing different patterns of response, depending on need. These messages are delivered by chemicals called neurotransmitters. Some transmitters excite the area of brain they serve, others dampen activity. The same chemical in a different site in the brain can have an opposite effect. These chemical neurotransmitters are released in discrete amounts from granules or storage units within the nerve cells. The granules are triggered to release their contents when the nerve cell has been appropriately stimulated.

What brain chemicals are involved in depression?

We now know there are over forty different types of neuro-transmitters (Fig 3.1). There are three neurotransmitter systems in the central nervous system (CNS) that are affected by anti-depressants:

- noradrenaline (NA)
- dopamine
- serotonin (5-hydroxytryptamine or 5-HT)

Noradrenaline is the key chemical in controlling the state of activity in the brain. In depressive illness, there is a change in the nerve cell receptors and this causes a slowing down of the release of NA at the cell synapse. The whole system becomes run down and less active.

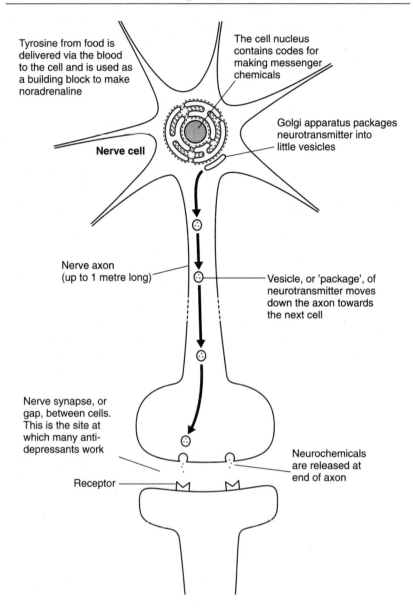

Tyrosine from food is delivered via the blood to the cell and is used as a building block to make noradrenaline

The cell nucleus contains codes for making messenger chemicals

Golgi apparatus packages neurotransmitter into little vesicles

Nerve cell

Nerve axon (up to 1 metre long)

Vesicle, or 'package', of neurotransmitter moves down the axon towards the next cell

Nerve synapse, or gap, between cells. This is the site at which many anti-depressants work

Neurochemicals are released at end of axon

Receptor

Fig 3.1 How neurotransmitters work

Tyrosine is a building block for the neurotransmitters noradrenaline and dopamine. Tyrosine can be found in food and is absorbed through the gut into the blood stream. It is then transported to the brain and pumped into nerve cells.

An enzyme works on the tyrosine to make *dopa,* and a second enzyme changes the dopa to *dopamine.* The third step converts dopamine to NA. The final product is stored in granules or vesicles in the nerve cells. The vesicles are released when the nerve is stimulated.

Serotonin (5-HT) is produced by enzymes from a chemical called *tryptophan.* Tryptophan in the blood is transported into serotonin nerve cells, where the tryptophan is converted into 5-HT by a series of chemical changes. The 5-HT made is stored in the nerve cell until the appropriate impulse arrives and the substance is released.

5-HT is made in specialised parts of the pons and medulla, structures in the mid-brain. Nerve cells spread out from these areas into the cortex or surface of the brain, the spinal cord and the specialised part of the brain called the limbic system. 5-HT is a key chemical in maintaining very basic and important animal responses. It helps control the cycles of liveliness and sleep. It is very important in producing aggression (a basic survival need), and also maintaining background mood.

Where do my moods actually come from within my brain?

The part of your brain known as the limbic system is very important in the production and maintenance of mood.

This part of the brain forms the margin (or 'limbus') of the 'newest' – most recently evolved – part of the brain, the cortex. It is formed in the shape of a 'C' (Fig 3.2). It includes the hippocampus, the amygdala, parts of the hypothalamus and thalamus, the nucleus accumbens and the basal nucleus. The last two are important in the production of acetylcholine (a neurotransmitter substance). The limbic system is joined by the cingulate gyrus and the parahippocampal gyrus.

The limbic system works with many other brain systems. Neuroscientists suggest that if the limbic system function is decreased, depression results. If limbic system activity is increased, inappropriate elation of mood or mania results. If the limbic system is malfunctioning, psychotic illness can result. This is a momentous and exciting area of research.

The limbic system gives humans (and other higher animals) a way of coping with their environment, and other people and animals within that environment (Fig. 3.3). Very basic survival behaviours like eating, drinking and reproducing are driven by the limbic system. Other parts of the limbic system are involved in feelings and emotions. Yet other parts of the limbic system link information received from all our senses to our state within.

The hypothalamus, part of the limbic system, is a control centre – like a thermostat – which regulates the body's internal environment. One example of its many activities is the regulation of eating and drinking. That's why appetite disturbance can be part of depression.

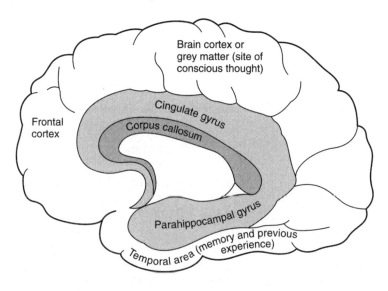

Fig 3.2 A cross-section of the brain showing some parts of the limbic system – where moods arise

The limbic system is divided into two sub-systems.

- First there is the hippocampus and its connections. This maintains our attention, and the formation of memory. It receives processed information from all our senses (touch, smell, sight, taste, hearing).
- Secondly, the limbic system divides into the amygdala and its connections. This area links what our senses are telling us, and defines the feeling of anxiety (only when appropriate, we hope). It helps form emotional links with our sensations as they occur.

The sense of smell has major links with the limbic system, giving rise to powerful emotions with some smells. Memory can be very rapidly and powerfully triggered by a smell. The memory returns with the emotion felt at that time. In the animal kingdom, smells 'cue' not just memories; they are often vital to initiate mating. Scents are relatively unimportant in humans – although the perfume industry would tell us otherwise.

How can stress, social problems and unhappiness affect your brain chemistry?

For a long time, scientists have recognised that there must be more to depression than the monoamine theory (see above). The brain chemistry of depressive illness realistically needs to explain, in chemical terms, the effect of early experiences (such as the loss of a parent), the effect of stress (such as abuse), and the social factors that are implicated in depression. Genetics too are involved.

There is now evidence from animal research that anti-depressants, given over some time, increase the production of 'neuroprotective proteins'. These substances occur naturally and are important in the growth and normal functioning of nerve cells. Antidepressant treatment activates the system that triggers so-called transcription substances. These control the expression of some genes in brain cells. Levels of this substance, called brain-derived neurotrophic factor (BDNF), are increased in the hippocampus.

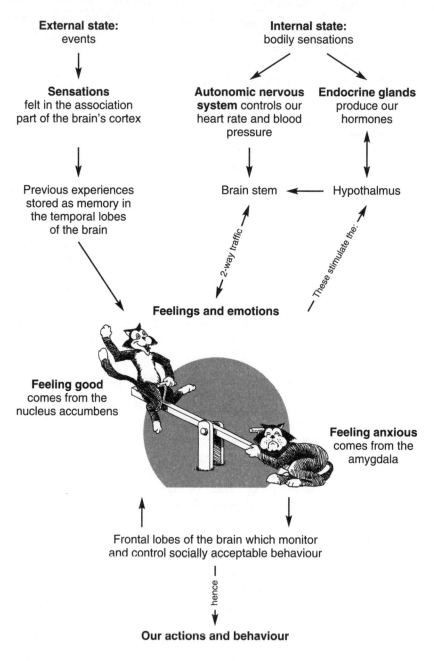

External state:
events

Sensations
felt in the association
part of the brain's cortex

Previous experiences
stored as memory in
the temporal lobes
of the brain

Internal state:
bodily sensations

**Autonomic nervous
system** controls our
heart rate and blood
pressure

Endocrine glands
produce our
hormones

Brain stem ← Hypothalmus

2-way traffic

These stimulate the:

Feelings and emotions

Feeling good
comes from the
nucleus accumbens

Feeling anxious
comes from the
amygdala

Frontal lobes of the brain which monitor
and control socially acceptable behaviour

hence

Our actions and behaviour

Fig 3.3 The brain's limbic system

BDNF belongs to a group of growth factors that help control nerve cell activities, ranging from the differentiation (or specialisation) of cells, to keeping the cells alive, once the brain is developed. It has been shown that, if experimental animals are stressed, there is a decrease in the amount of BDNF in the hippocampus. This effect is opposed, or counteracted by, anti-depressant treatment. It seems that stress 'down-regulates' or dampens, the expression of the substance that helps maintain lively healthy brain cells.

There is some evidence that chronic severe depression causes some atrophy or shrinkage in the hippocampus. Depressive illness could therefore be seen as a very subtle form of degeneration in some nerve cells. Protective substances like BDNF might act to reverse this effect. We know, too, that electroconvulsive therapy (ECT) helps promote the BDNF and can induce positive, regenerative changes within the hippocampus.

So can the brain alter itself when you are stressed or depressed?

We used to think that the brain could never regenerate itself. We now know that neurones are generated throughout life, and that parts of the brain are 'plastic' or capable of change. The hippocampal cells' vitality may be influenced by many elements, including genetic influences, raised steroid levels (as occurs in stress), some viral infections, lack of oxygen, low blood sugar levels, and psychologically stressful events. Antidepressants are thought to protect against this damage.

BDNF not only determines whether some nerve cells live or die. It also regulates the networks that nerve cells make with each other. BDNF can strengthen, or can dampen down, nerve connections. Changes in the patterns of connections between nerve cells help form memory, and determine responses to stress. It allows the brain to be 'plastic' or malleable in its responses to the environment, so forming new patterns of response as required. These same mechanisms happen in the amygdala, and can produce fear responses when necessary.

Stresses may actually *change* these connecting patterns. This may go some way to explain the thinking, and emotional changes that occur in mood disorders. Antidepressants magnify nerve synapse connecting ability. It is likely that different antidepressants affect synapse connectivity in subtly different ways.

The picture is yet more complicated. Within the hippocampus, there are two types (1 and 2) of steroid receptors. These are very important in producing the body's response to stress. Chemicals that are type 2 antagonists (i.e. work against them), have been shown to protect against the changes that would otherwise happen in the nerve endings of experimental animals who have been stressed. These substances are currently being researched as possible future antidepressant agents.

There is increasing evidence that early experience of stress can damage the hippocampus. If young rats are repeatedly separated from their mothers, changes in nerve connections in the hippocampus can be seen (they become less adaptable). We are now gathering evidence that early psychological trauma and abuse causes permanent damage – something we have known instinctively for a very long time.

A simpler explanation

Can you explain to me in simple terms why I'm depressed. What's actually happening to me?

There are various ways of understanding depression. You can explain it in terms of brain chemistry, of genetics, of people's life circumstances. Sometimes it seems a natural response to what's happened to you, sometimes it seems like a bolt from the blue, and we are still a long way from understanding everything about how the brain works.

Many people don't seem to want a detailed explanation of the changes in brain chemistry, of the depletion of neurotransmitters that we find associated with depression. Of course that's useful if you want to know exactly why antidepressants help, but we can use motorcars or computers for a much simpler explanation.

It's as if people with depression have flat batteries. They've had too many demands on their circuits, not enough chance to recharge themselves, and they can't start their motor one cold damp morning. Taking antidepressants is like having your battery charged up; it takes some time to recharge. (That's why a full course of antidepressants takes some months.) When your battery is charged up, you can start your own engine, go for a good drive, and keep it topped up by taking care of it. That's why looking after yourself – proper maintenance and recreation (i.e. re-creation) – is so important.

For computer experts, the analogy is that you've had too much data coming in and your hard drive is full of chaotic randomly stored stuff. You can't process any more information, then the system becomes erratic, your usual programmes don't work so well. You start getting error messages, and finally the whole thing crashes while you're trying to do something important. Perhaps, counselling or psychotherapy is like defragmenting your hard drive, a process of tidying up untidy memories and thoughts to free up storage space so that you can cope with today's activity, and, yes, we do have Helplines for humans (for example, the Samaritans – see Appendix 1) as well as for computers.

Actually the human brain is still light years more complex than our fastest computers, so these analogies have their limitations, but we can still use these devices without understanding a complicated explanation of their mechanisms!

Another model is a rather more philosophical one: people with depression have come to feel that they're trapped; they've lost sight of the light at the end of the tunnel; they have lost the freedom of choice, and the control over their lives that we all need. Reminding ourselves that we always do have choice in our lives and starting to make some choices – however simple – can be a good start. (That's why painting the kitchen ceiling or having your hair done can be good therapy.)

Some psychological theories of depression

Psychoanalytical theory

Sigmund Freud noted how similar mourning and grieving and depression are. Depression could be a response to loss.

The loss may be a bereavement, a separation, redundancy, bankruptcy, loss of a home. Depression can also be caused by a threatened loss – perhaps loss of health and independence, the threat of job loss, the threat of a broken marriage. You do not need to be trained in psychoanalysis to see how very persuasive this theory is.

Learning theory

This was put forward by the psychologist Seligman. He found that, if he reared rats who had little or no control over their environment, they are poor at getting out of bad situations – even when given an opportunity to escape, they do not take it. They have learnt that their behaviours, and what happens to them, are not linked. Failure leads to a feeling of helplessness and a belief that whatever you do will not change anything – this can become a starting point for depressive thinking.

Cognitive theory

This puts forward the idea that if you are repeatedly negative, you can unknowingly build up a depressive way of dealing with life, which can go on to make you ill. The negativity becomes a self-fulfilling prophecy. This view can be challenged with cognitive behaviour therapy (see Chapter 5).

Social factors

There are certain social factors that seem to make people more vulnerable to depression. They make up an unfavourable background in which illness is more easily provoked. Studies were done by Brown, a sociologist, looking at a group of inner city young women who became depressed. Those who became ill tended to be unemployed outside the home; had no intimate, confiding relationship; had three or more children under the age of 14 at home, and had lost their mother before they were aged 11. Low self-esteem was later found to make the women more vulnerable. Having a low income was also a valid factor. To this list was added the occurrence of threatening life-events, or serious difficulties (see below).

Life-events

These are not the small day-by-day happenings but bigger events that require us to adapt and change to cope with them. A new baby may be a total joy, and much wanted, but will require both parents to make huge changes in their lives to accommodate the event. Changes cause stress, and stress can go on to cause mood shifts. Promotion may be exciting, but it also can be stressful. Other life-events are more clearly stress-provoking, such as the loss of a job or marital breakdown.

You are more likely to become depressed if there has been a cluster of life-events in the preceding 6–12 months than if your life has been settled.

Physical illness and depression

Depression can occur as part of a wide range of illnesses and physical factors. The following box is long but is not in any way inclusive. It just shows some of the causes. Do not be alarmed. It is relatively unusual for there to be a physical underlying cause for depression – it is much more often psychological factors, stresses and genetics that are responsible for depressive illness.

Box 3.1 Illnesses and other factors causing depression

Endocrine (gland) dysfunction	over- or underactive thyroid gland over- or underactive adrenal gland
Kidney disease	kidney failure and renal dialysis
Infections	'flu glandular fever hepatitis shingles

Anaemia	folate deficiency
	iron deficiency (the most common)
	pernicious anaemia
	    (vitamin B_{12} deficiency)
	(both pernicious anaemia and folate
	    deficiency occur in alcoholism)

Neurological, brain disease	dementia epilepsy multiple sclerosis Parkinson's disease stroke
Stopping drugs	alcohol (withdrawal or use of) amphetamines benzodiazepines (Valium family)
Malignant disease	brain tumour cancer of the pancreas lung cancer
Side-effect of drug treatment	anti-epileptic drugs barbiturates (phenobarbitone) beta-blockers chemotherapy (anticancer treatment) interferon L-dopa (used for the treatment of Parkinson's disease) methyldopa (Aldomet) most tranquillisers and sleeping tablets Roaccutane (for severe acne) steroids (prednisolone)

Depression and dementia

Dementia means a persistent overall decline in all mental abilities (memory, intellect and personality) without any kind of loss of consciousness. It is usually a slow process. Dementia can sometimes be confused with depression: the two illnesses can co-exist, or each can look like the other in isolation.

Depression commonly causes decreased concentration, and this can look like poor memory functioning. If you are unable to concentrate, you do not take the information in for storage, and it is not there for retrieval later – your memory will seem poor. In about two-thirds of elderly depressed people there are signs of memory difficulties if they are very carefully tested. If these difficulties are very marked, they can look exceedingly like someone who is dementing. However, when the depression is treated, the 'dementia' goes completely, memory and concentration return. This phenomenon is called pseudodementia.

The opposite situation can occur. People who are beginning to function less well, and are in the process of developing a dementing illness, can become depressed. This may be because they can see what is happening, and become depressed. Occasionally – especially if they are depressed for the first time in late life – this can be a part of the dementing illness itself. Whatever the situation, if an elderly person is clinically depressed, plus or minus dementia, they need vigorous treatment.

Even in advanced dementia, depression can be treated and treatment will often improve the quality of life significantly. Antidepressant medication needs to be chosen with more care in the elderly, because they have more problems with side-effects. Antidepressants certainly work well in the elderly – there are no age bars. Electroconvulsive therapy (ECT) can also be used in the elderly to very good effect. ECT may in fact be a safer option than some complicated regimens of medication. Somebody who is suffering from dementia and depression will not have their dementia worsened by ECT.

Epilepsy

My son was diagnosed as having epilepsy six months ago and was put on to an anti-epileptic drug. He has slowed down and become depressed. Could this be due to his medication?

The diagnosis of epilepsy has major implications for anybody, and there is the added indignity of being unable to drive a motor vehicle until free of seizures for a year. Epilepsy is still, unfortunately, treated as a stigmatising condition and it causes unpredictable and often extremely embarrassing loss of control. No wonder this young man is feeling down.

In addition, a number of the older antiepileptic drugs (AEDs), whilst not causing clinical depression, can result in mental slowing, fatigue and reduction in liveliness. The AEDs most likely to do this are phenytoin (Epanutin) and phenobarbitone, but almost all AEDs can cause these problems in a small proportion of individuals. It is generally best, in order to avoid these adverse effects as far as possible, to build up the dosage slowly and generally to use newer AEDs like lamotrigine, although carbamazepine and sodium valproate are well tried and tested AEDs with relatively few adverse effects.

When epilepsy is diagnosed, the individual and their family are likely to need a lot of support and information about the condition. However, over 50% of people will be completely controlled on one AED and about 30% can stop medication after 4–5 years.

Antidepressants nearly all have some tendency to make epilepsy worse; generally this is not a particularly important consideration when compared with the necessity of treating the depression. At times seizure control is improved by lifting the mood. ECT may be indicated in cases of severe depression in someone with epilepsy.

Depression and learning disability

Some degree of learning disability is present in 2–3% of the population, and a quarter of these people show evidence of psychiatric disorder. This increased rate of psychiatric illness might be partly due to psychological factors, which include the stigma of being learning disabled, and the frustrations and limitations of daily life. It may also partly be due to altered brain functioning (which has given rise to the learning disability).

In people with learning disabilities, depression is much more likely to show itself with changes in behaviour rather than the person actually complaining of feeling depressed. Agitation and overactivity can occur, but withdrawn behaviour is especially likely. Apathy and general slowing down are very common. Sometimes repetitive and compulsive behaviour may emerge. Sometimes the depression may show itself by the development of physical symptoms as a sign of distress (somatisation).

It is very important to identify depression in people with learning disabilities because, if missed, the depression may cause a quite marked decline in ability to cope, and this, of course, is responsible for a great deal of misery and a poorer quality of life.

Multiple sclerosis

Multiple sclerosis causes isolated patches of damage to myelin (the covering of long nerve axons). A scar results, and later the nerve axon is damaged. It is one of the most common diseases of the nervous system in temperate climates. It affects the central nervous system and causes an enormous variety of symptoms and signs. There is a tendency to remission and relapse. It can be a relatively benign disease. For others, there is a poorer prognosis.

Psychiatric symptoms, especially anxiety and depression, are found in about 40% of people with multiple sclerosis while they are in remission, and in about 90% when they are in an active phase of the illness. Their symptoms may be very mild to severe.

In one study, the degree of psychiatric difficulty was found to be related to the amount of social stresses present at that time. The vulnerability to psychiatric illness, brought about by the multiple sclerosis, seemed to increase the harmful effect of stress in the environment – it acts as a magnifying agent. Psychiatric illness in multiple sclerosis should not be seen as an inevitable or untreatable part of the illness. It is as amenable to treatment as depression caused by any other cause. It is always essential to treat depression in these circumstances, since somebody who is disabled and depressed is far more incapacitated than someone who is disabled with a normal mood.

Parkinson's disease

Parkinson's disease is a disease in which there is a falling off of the numbers of nerve cells in the pigmented cells (substantia nigra) in the brain stem. The cause is unknown in most people, although very rarely poisons, such as carbon monoxide or repeated head injury (as in punch-drunk syndrome), are responsible. Parkinson's disease is characterised by a muscular tremor, muscular stiffness and slowing of movement. In addition, some sort of mental changes can be seen in up to 40% of people with Parkinson's disease.

Depression occurs in about a third of people with Parkinson's disease – this is not merely a reaction to the diagnosis, or the disability, but is perhaps an integral part of the illness process affecting the brain. It has been suggested that a decrease in brain 5-HT and noradrenaline, which occurs in Parkinson's disease, can lead on to depression.

The depression that occurs in Parkinson's disease is usually mild to moderate in its intensity. It responds to the same sort of treatment as any other depressive illness, but the older anti-depressants can sometimes cause a seeming worsening in the movement disorder (as a side-effect). This is removed if the drug is stopped. Newer antidepressants, such as fluoxetine (Prozac), can be easier to tolerate in Parkinson's disease and can be very effective indeed. In severe depression and Parkinson's disease, ECT (electroconvulsive therapy) can be used to very good effect. There may even be a temporary improvement in the symptoms of Parkinson's disease with this treatment. Unfortunately, this improvement is not sustained.

Stroke

Depression is common after strokes – maybe 40% of people who have a stroke will become clinically depressed. Losing the use of part of one's body is such a catastrophic, frustrating event, with the addition of possible loss of job, income, plans for the future, hobbies and social interests. The depressive illness may also be seen as part of the brain's response to the damage caused by the stroke.

So people recovering from strokes can certainly get depressed. It is essential that depression following stroke is treated vigorously – not least because recovery would otherwise be significantly delayed. Remember that depression can be contagious, and the close family of someone with depression can also become depressed. If you are a carer, don't overlook your own needs. You are pretty indispensable, so look after yourself too, and discuss how you feel with your own doctor.

Trauma

My husband came off his motorbike 3 months ago. He was knocked out for a few minutes. He went to the Casualty Department and they said his X-ray was normal. However, he has not got back to his old self and is tired all the time. He can't cope at work. Could this be depression?

Anybody who has been knocked out, even very briefly, is likely to have a period of fatigue sometimes for up to 6 months. Knockout blows are not as benign as they seem in films. A blow that is sufficiently severe to impair consciousness is likely also to have disrupted the deeper regions of the brain as it is swirled about in the skull. The brain has a jelly-like consistency and is attached to the rest of the nervous system by a central stalk, which contains the nerve centres controlling alertness. If these are shaken up (as is usually the case in head injury), fatigue results. The usual process after head injury of this kind is for headache to be prominent at first, often with dizziness (as the balance organs are often also disrupted). Then fatigue, poor concentration and irritability occur.

It is vital to be aware of all this so that your husband does not return to work too soon, as this will tend to exacerbate the fatigue and reduce his confidence. Careful support and understanding on your part and that of your family and his employers is very important. Return to work should be gradual, but may well take up to 6 months. This is not usually evidence of depression, but may lead on to that, if recovery is slow or misunderstood, and he starts to lose hope, expecting to be ill – even brain damaged – when this is not the case. The vast majority of people with a brief loss of consciousness or a post-traumatic amnesia of less than 24 hours (inability to remember events from the time of the accident) will return to their normal selves, but slowly, over a course of up to 6 months.

Other medication and depression

I'm on lots of tablets for other health problems, and I've been getting very depressed. Could any of my other medication actually cause depression?

Yes, they certainly could. One way of checking if any of your other treatment could be affecting your mood is by reading the (very) small print on the slips that come with your medication. Don't be put off by the long lists of possible side-effects, as most of these are actually quite rare. Your chemist or your GP would be a good person to ask whether depression is a possible side-effect of any particular medication.

Some drugs that are well recognised as affecting your mood were listed earlier in Box 3.1, but this list is not exhaustive.

Chronic illness can in itself be depressing. Poor pain control (from a slipped disc or arthritis, for example) is very debilitating. Loss of mobility (say from a broken leg or a stroke) causes loss of social contacts and recreation. Recovery from major surgery can also be an exhausting business. Some medical treatments used can also make you depressed.

Does the Pill make you depressed?

Almost certainly not, although some women do seem to be particularly sensitive to the effects of the oestrogen in the combined oral contraceptive pill, and may feel more moody or irritable. Trying a different combination pill often seems to do the trick. Switching to a brand with a lower dose of oestrogen may help. If that fails, consider using the progestogen-only pill (POP). Remember this has to be taken more carefully at the same time every day, and does have a failure rate of about 1% per year (that means that 1 in 100 women using this method of contraception will become pregnant in a year). The depot-contraceptive injection, Depo-Provera, works in the same way, has a similar failure rate, and also has no oestrogen in it.

If you are going through a bad spell, or are feeling unsettled, it's really important not to overlook safe contraception. People who are depressed may not place enough value on looking after themselves, and may take risks that they wouldn't usually consider. You certainly don't want to have to be thinking about dealing with an unexpected pregnancy when you're depressed.

As we have seen, there are a multitude of causes and factors that bring about depressive illness. The causes in one person are never the same in someone else – we each have our own story and our unique background, which will colour our illness.

4
Self-help

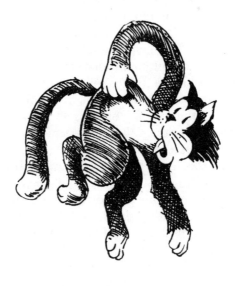

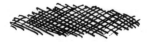

We all have our own ways of dealing with depression. Here's a list we've compiled from our patients, from our families and friends, from books, pamphlets, the Internet, and from just plain common-sense. Some of these answers won't be right for you, some could be excellent. Suggestions are divided into the following sections:

- at home
- at work
- with other people
- at night.

Look through these and try some until you find something useful. At the end we list some self-help tactics for early signs of mania.

At home

General

- If you are stuck, try to choose basic activities that you know you can do, not major challenges, which would be difficult at the best of times.
- In India they have laughing clubs. Try it on your own. Laughing, if you can, does help.
- If you're feeling bogged down, and everyone you know seems to irritate you, try to spend time among people you don't know, who won't be intrusive. Sometimes it's easier to confide in a neutral stranger.
- Take one bit of the day at a time, perhaps just until lunch or tea time. Don't think too far ahead. (One whole day at a time may seem too much.)
- Just for the time being, put your emotional problems on hold. Get back into them later on when you recover. Try to visualise the problem being put in a box that you have put on a shelf to deal with later. It will keep it confined, but not forgotten.
- Forgive yourself. Remind yourself that you are not a bad person.
- Keep a diary. Write it down. Get it out on paper. Defining it with pen and ink may help you stop dwelling on it and move on. If it's really bad stuff, writing it out and then destroying it can sometimes help.

Hobbies

- Music helps many people. Really listen to music, both old favourites and something new.

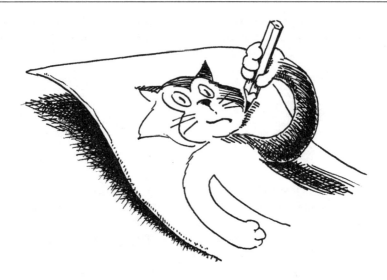

- Reading is good. If you can't concentrate on something
  serious escape into something lighthearted. It doesn't
  matter whether it's pulp fiction, Harry Potter or P.G.
  Wodehouse. Don't tackle anything too gloomy until you're
  strong enough for it: Dostoevsky isn't a good idea when
  you're feeling low. Re-reading a favourite book can be like
  meeting an old friend. If your concentration is poor,
  knowing the plot already will make the read easier.
- Put a silly game on the computer, but not all night.
- Mess about in the garden. Plant something if the weather
  permits; and then you can look after it and watch it grow, a
  curiously satisfying experience. Pot plants indoors can be
  equally rewarding.

Relaxation

- Take a long bath by candlelight. Get some of those soothing
  scented bathroom candles.
- Get a really funny classic video out. Allow yourself to have
  a good laugh watching it.
- Sing along to your favourite record – even if you're tone

deaf! Sing in your car if you don't want to make too much
noise at home. Singing uses your chest and diaphragmatic
muscles, gets your circulation going, blows away the
cobwebs, and is surprisingly relaxing.
* Find out how to meditate. Evening classes are often run by
  local authorities. If you are feeling too low to meditate,
  read something out loud.
* Concentrate on enjoying the comic strip in your newspaper,
  leave the serious stuff for later. There's enough sadness in
  the world.

Exercise

* Get some exercise. Go to the gym, walk, run or cycle. Do it
  every day, just for 20 minutes is a good start. Don't take it
  too seriously, just try to get out of breath a little.
* Practice dancing. Start off on your own. It doesn't matter if
  you aren't too elegant – who's looking anyway?
* Set yourself a small task, such as an easy piece of
  housework – perhaps clearing out an old cupboard – and
  actually do it. Enjoy the feeling of accomplishment. Then
  do a slightly larger task. Paint the kitchen ceiling, or clear
  out the garden shed.
* Springclean (even if it's the autumn). Get rid of a box full
  of stuff that you know you'll never use or wear again. Give
  it to a charity shop, or put it out for recycling. Then stand
  back, admire the space you've cleared, and enjoy the
  feeling that somebody else will benefit from your donation.

Diet

* Look after your nutrition. Eat regularly and properly –
  sometimes it's easier to eat little and often. Don't stuff
  yourself with comfort food, but allow yourself an
  occasional treat – even if it is junk food. Cheat sometimes –
  have a ready meal to save time and bother.

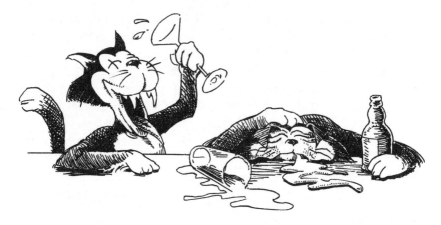

- Be careful about alcohol. Drinking heavily or regularly makes depression worse. Antidepressants can also alter how a drink will affect you. Antidepressants cannot work effectively if you are drinking anything more than just modest amounts.
- Cook yourself a special recipe. Next time, ask a friend to join you.

Treats

- Treats are very important! Give yourself a treat: buy yourself something you like. The treat does not have to be costly – a special soap or shampoo can be a treat.
- Be a bit special for a while – look after yourself more. Don't take yourself for granted.
- Chocolate is rumoured to have a mild antidepressant effect. Perhaps this could one of your treats.
- Buy yourself some flowers.

Getting help

- If things are really bad and you feel like harming yourself in some way, don't be on your own. Make sure there are other people around. Make human contact, by phone if not in person. If you haven't got anyone you can phone, use the

Samaritans (see Appendix 1); they are not professional counsellors but they are there to help.
- Keep in touch with your doctor. Work with him or her. Don't miss appointments, even if you feel too tired or ill to go. If you feel you aren't making progress or getting anywhere, say so. Ask for further help, maybe a medication review or a further opinion. If you are not progressing adequately, this is nobody's fault; the problem needs to be addressed.

If you are on medication:
- Take it consistently (the same time each day) and persistently (for as long as directed).
- Find out from your GP what side-effects may occur, and what to do if they do.
- Don't stop taking medication or change dosage without taking your doctor's advice.
- Ask about mixing medication. If you need to take anything else (even cold remedies – these can interact with some antidepressants), ask your chemist or GP. Ask about alcohol if you need to.

At work

- Always try to avoid sitting at your desk for meal breaks and coffee. Go and mix with other people, or just get some fresh air and private space somewhere.
- Let people know that you're not 100% at the moment. Confide in someone, get someone on your side. Can any part of your work be eased, put on the back burner for the time being?
- When you are feeling depressed, you may find that you can't manage your usual amount of mental work, but you probably can do more physical activities instead (even if you don't really want to much). Try to put off the more challenging, intellectual work until you are feeling better.

- Don't tackle difficult tasks when you are down. Avoid major work or personal decisions. Delegate, shelve or pass on as much responsibility as you can, try to concentrate on the routine – which can be surprisingly soothing and much more easily achievable.
- Use time management tactics. Pace yourself, divide your work into smaller chunks, and work at a steady pace. Don't rush, take it piece by piece. Prioritise your tasks, and be prepared to abandon some of your lower priorities – or shelve some of your more overwhelming tasks. If you find that you are a procrastinator, start by getting one thing done at a time. Make a list of things you need to do and divide them up into:

  - Do it now, i.e. today's jobs (keep this list short)
  - Do it later, and put these in your diary
  - Get someone else to do it (if you can)
  - Bin it (and be ruthless).

- Beware 'displacement activity', for example making yourself frightfully busy with something unimportant.
- Cross the things that you've achieved off the list, but check through them occasionally. Give yourself a pat on the back about the ones you've done. This works at home or at work.
- If you have an Occupational Health Department, let them know if you are not well. They are an independent source of advice and may be able to help make adjustments to your workplace to reduce the pressure until things improve.
- Look forward to a target to get through the week, e.g. going out to eat with friends on a Friday night.
- Be realistic. Don't demand too much from yourself or set yourself impossible tasks that you are not going to manage, as they will only increase feelings of failure and hopelessness.
- Make time for yourself in your working day.
- Don't be a perfectionist. Settle for 'good enough' just for the time being. Setting too high a target is very annihilating!

With other people

- Being with other people is better than being on your own.
- Pay someone a compliment unexpectedly.
- Phone friends for a chat.
- Confront your fears. If you're avoiding something, perhaps feeling guilty about it, ask a friend to help see you through it, or think of something else you want to do even less, and do the first thing instead! (You have to creep up on your fears sometimes.)
- Do something for someone else. Find out about voluntary work. It can help you start to think more about other people and focus rather less about yourself. There's always someone who is in a worse situation than yourself. Putting something back in for someone else always helps.
- Ignore well-meaning advice to 'pull yourself together'. Depression is an illness, and recovery usually requires antidepressant therapy and/or psychotherapy. You cannot make yourself 'snap out' of depression any more than you can ignore appendicitis, but you can decide to tackle it, to deal with it, and to get help to sort it out.
- Don't neglect your social life. Keep in touch with friends, as they can recharge your batteries too. A brief postcard to tell someone that you are thinking of them can be a delight to receive, and may be easier to do. Speaking on the telephone can be difficult when you are depressed.

At night

Sleep is vital and the best remedy.

- Don't wind yourself up at night with too much late TV.
- Get off the computer. The light from the screen will alert you and may interfere with sleep.
- Watch the sunset, the moon, the stars, or the sunrise.

- Don't lie in bed all day. The more you feel like staying in bed, the more you should resist it. Your body needs to be physically active to keep your body clock and natural body rhythms running. The more you lie in bed the less you'll get done. If you feel too tired to stand up, get out of bed and stagger into a warm bath straight away. This will gently get you going and help you get started on the day ahead. Depression reduces your drive, but beware the vicious circle of staying in bed and then feeling guilty about being slothful. This just makes depression worse. Depression is often worse in the mornings – but it does *not* ease by staying in bed. You need to be up, and distracted from your thoughts.
- Try to keep your body clock running at the right time – don't turn night into day.
- If you are going through a bad patch of early morning waking (perhaps at 3–4 am) and cannot get back to sleep, get up and let your mind occupy itself with something other than fretting over your worries. Don't lie there worrying about not sleeping. Read, write a letter, have a warm drink (but no caffeine or alcohol), tidy up your desk. Putting things into place physically may help your mind wind down and stop it bothering the rest of you. Although losing some sleep temporarily is unpleasant, you won't become ill because of it.
- Do not accept negative thoughts. Identify them and resist them. They are a very insidious part of depression. These irrational, unpleasant thoughts will disappear when your treatment kicks in. Recognise these thoughts for what they are and think up some distractions from them. Everyone has horrid thoughts at some time and these get exaggerated when your defences are down. If negative thoughts start to include thinking that things would be better if you were dead and you start to think about self-harm or suicide a lot, tell your doctor. If you feel bad in the night and you are reluctant to phone the GP, remember the Samaritans are on duty all night, as are the staff in the local Accident and Emergency department. NHS Direct (0845 4647)

is a 24-hour advice line staffed by experienced health professionals who can give valuable advice and support.

- Suicide is irreversible – don't act on your unrealistically hopeless thoughts. Treatment makes these thoughts, ideas and impulses go away. Feeling that nothing helps and that things are hopeless is part of the illness. Try to separate the real you from these irrational thoughts. They will then bother you less.
- Use earplugs if your bedroom is noisy.
- Eat early, so that your digestion has settled down before you go to bed.
- Avoid late caffeine or alcohol. Alcohol isn't a good sleeping draught as you tend to wake up when it wears off at 2–3 in the morning, with a hangover and needing to spend a penny.
- Hot milky drinks seem to help.
- Make sure that your bedroom is quiet and comfortable, not too hot and stuffy, nor too cold.
- Have a consistent routine of going to bed at the same time, not too late, and read or listen to the radio to settle yourself down.
- Don't get overtired. A bit of fresh air and an evening walk can relax your tired muscles.
- Avoid daytime naps if you are not sleeping well at night. If you do need a nap, do this after lunch and put the alarm clock on for, say, 1½ hours later.
- Treat yourself to nice fresh pyjamas and sheets. Is your bed comfortable?
- Music playing in the background can be a pleasant distraction from bothersome intrusive thoughts when you are settling down at night.
- Try learning a simple relaxing exercise. Try to regularise your breathing to be slower and deeper while you think of a favourite place – visualise the scene and enjoy it. Yoga classes teach this method.

Self-help tactics for early signs of mania

Signs of going high or hypomanic may include the following:

- broken sleep
- early waking
- overactivity with lots of grandiose ideas and plans
- reduced concentration
- selfishness, loss of usual consideration for others
- impatience and irritability
- loads of energy
- increased spending
- unwise or indiscreet decisions
- rapid speech
- loss of usual inhibitions, with promiscuity or increase in
  alcohol use.

The excitement of mania feeds on itself and leads to an increasingly hectic mood spiral, progressively detaching you from life's realities. So, to calm yourself down:

General

- Switch off from any major decisions, life plans or big
  purchases. Try to wait until you are more settled.
- Actively reduce your work commitments; leave the crucial
  stuff for another time.
- Plan out your day to avoid rushing. Aim to achieve the bare
  minimum.
- Be particularly careful when driving, especially if you are
  on any medication.
- Be particularly careful not to be tactless with friends and
  relatives – you will need them later.
- Switch from caffeine-containing drinks to herbal teas.
- Don't use alcohol as a stimulant, and avoid street drugs
  totally.

- Don't stay up watching the late TV shows; they'll wind you up more.
- Switch off the computer in the evening; don't get excited by surfing the net at night.
- Discuss any medication that you are taking with your doctor; some can induce mania.
- Discuss using a suitable tranquilliser with your doctor. Drugs such as haloperidol or chlorpromazine are often helpful, and you may need only a small dose for some days, if you act quickly enough.
- Avoid late parties, or exciting outings.
- Get your feet back on the ground, remind yourself that you are at risk of getting yourself into trouble at the moment, that you will later have to clear up.
- Concentrate your thoughts, not on your latest exciting schemes but on boring matter of fact things. Sorting out bills and housework can be good ways of bringing yourself down to earth.
- Slow down. Walk, talk and think more slowly.
- If you are getting grandiose fantasies about yourself, deflate these by repeatedly saying, 'I'm just Joe Bloggs' or 'It's only me really; I'm not Superman or Superwoman.'
- Try and ask for help early. Mood can rapidly become less manageable – later on you may be too ill to recognise it.

Sort out your sleep

- People with bipolar disorder are especially vulnerable when sleep-deprived.
- Get plenty of exercise in the day to relax yourself.
- Be prepared to use some night medication, herbal or prescribed, for short periods.
- If you do wake early full of ideas, don't get up but stay put, and plan how to reduce the pressure in the day ahead.

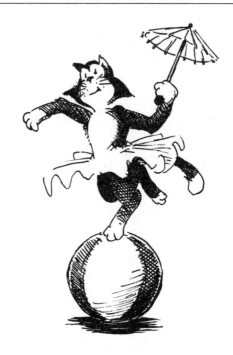

Apart from mood stabilising drugs how can I help myself stay level? Is there anything I can do to manage myself better?

Moods don't usually go out of control overnight. You usually have some warning of a mood swing, but being aware of your current mood level is not always easy. Quite often you don't realise you are irritable until after you've snapped at someone. Learning to recognise your own early warning signals of a downswing into depression or an upswing into hypomania can give you the chance to catch it early and prevent things going very wrong.

If you can easily recognise signs of trouble, one approach is to ask your doctor for a small supply of medication to use at the earliest sign of trouble. This can be both reassuring (you have the means to help yourself rapidly) and very effective.

5

Treatment of depression

Most people with depression can be successfully treated by their GPs. A minority – maybe 5% – may need to see a psychiatrist, and most of these people will be treated as outpatients. Treatment of depression involves medication, 'talking treatment' (psychological therapies, e.g. counselling and psychotherapy), or a combination of both.

Depression may pass unrecognised by sufferers, who put up with the loss of energy, anxiety, poor sleep, low moods, and sexual difficulties. It makes a sufferer think that it is just part of life. Untreated depression leads to much misery and ill health – sadly, even loss of life. It is so important that depression is fully and adequately treated. Nobody wants to take medication unless necessary, but medication plays a key part in most people's treatment.

A wide variety of antidepressant drugs is available. We describe the range of drugs and their side-effects. Antidepressants are not addictive. Treatment with these drugs needs to continue for a number of months – usually at least 6 months from when you start to feel better. It can take up to 3 weeks for these drugs to work, although many people notice improved sleep and more stable mood within the first week.

Depression also lowers your self-esteem, and time spent with a sympathetic counsellor or therapist can help you start to repair this damage. Counsellors and psychotherapists are available in many – but not all – GP surgeries, as well as in day hospitals, Community Mental Health Teams, and in the private sector. We discuss the different types of 'talking treatments' available, including one-to-one therapy, self-help group therapy, and therapies such as Cognitive Behavioural Therapy, for which there is good evidence of effectiveness.

Choosing your doctor

How can I choose a GP who will really understand depression?

GPs in the UK all undergo vocational training, which includes assessing ability to deal with psychological aspects of illness, so all GPs will have plenty of experience in dealing with depression – it's part of everyday work. Most GPs work in groups nowadays (there is a minority of single-handed GPs too, who give a personal one-to-one service), so you should be able to decide whether you prefer to see a male or female doctor, or an older or younger one. Start by asking among friends for personal recommendations. Most GPs aren't really in a position to offer detailed, in-depth counselling owing to time pressures, nor is that really appropriate when you're feeling very low.

Of course, we all have different chemistry, and nobody can guarantee that any two people will get on. See whether the practice has an attached counsellor, or can recommend good local ones. When you meet your GP, see if you are comfortable and whether you are going to be able to work with the doctor. You can always move to another practice if you really don't get on, but this should be a last resort. If you cannot find a doctor, the local health authority will allocate you one.

Few GPs actually have official further qualifications in psychiatric illness, so looking for letters after the name in the Medical Register or the Practice Profile (every practice has one), or on a practice website, is not so helpful.

Membership of the Royal College of GPs (MRCGP) does confirm that a GP has passed a thorough vetting in all aspects of family medicine, with special emphasis on psychological issues.

The most important part of a GP's job in dealing with someone who is depressed is assessment and starting medication when appropriate. So don't be too picky, and don't worry about shopping around for someone special. What's more important is entering into a working relationship with your GP, being able to trust that relationship, and making it work for you.

I don't get on with my GP. I need to talk about how depressed I feel, but she's not very sympathetic. What can I do?

It can be quite a skill to get the best out of your GP. Try thinking of them as a scarce resource that you need to work with well to get the best results. Some ways of doing this are to make early appointments rather than coming in with a complicated agenda at the end of a hectic surgery (this is likely to mean that you will be kept waiting less, too). Writing a list or letter can help you focus on what you actually want your GP to deal with. Be prepared to come again on a second occasion rather than go through a lengthy list when there are other people waiting.

Many (or all) NHS GPs are pretty hard pressed for time, but that shouldn't mean that they will not be interested in addressing emotional problems as well as sore throats and Pill prescriptions. All GPs are trained in looking in depth at psychological and social aspects of the problems. Every GP's training includes video sessions to help improve their consultation skills.

My GP never seems to have much time. How can I talk about depression to him?

The average GP appointment is about 10 minutes nowadays, and has become longer as we have more health promotion to insert into it. (That's advice on smoking, drinking, diet, exercise, BP checks and contraceptive advice.) Sometimes it seems as if there isn't time to tackle all this – 10 minutes does not sound much, but if you add it up it over a year it comes to 46 minutes on average per patient.

With a bit of leeway, most GPs normally make enough time to assess and treat depression in a busy surgery setting, but might use a series of short meetings to do this rather than one big one. Some people just need a prescription, so most of us find we can fit the occasional longer consultation into the working day, sufficient to assess and treat depression. Some GPs are rather 'counselling-orientated' and are able to engage in brief counselling themselves. Others will work with a counsellor, within the practice or known to them. People who are very depressed are not usually ready to do a lot of talking. It is best not to tackle painful issues until you are fit enough to deal with them – then talking can be very productive.

What constitutes good practice in medicine?

Of course there is still a wide range of choice of treatments for all conditions, and depression is no exception. Where problems arise with a treatment, if the doctor concerned has practised in line with 'a recognised body of medical opinion', the doctor will be unlikely to be considered negligent. If national guidelines have been published by NICE (National Institute for Clinical Excellence) or any other body, such as the Royal College of Psychiatrists or the Royal College of GPs, doctors can still practise outside them, but on their own responsibility.

All the drugs used in psychiatry today have been very extensively researched. Side-effects and interactions are well recognised. What is harder to do research into is the 'talking treatments', such as counselling and psychotherapy. These are costly resources and health authorities won't just take it for granted that they are beneficial. Those who want to provide counsellors in General Practices have had to argue the case very hard. Counselling is very popular with people, but its efficacy is debated.

Choosing your treatment

How do doctors decide which treatment is the best?

We are aware of good scientific evidence that treatments are effective and safe. This is by far the strongest and most objective reason, and we try increasingly nowadays to base medical treatment on published evidence. There are many medical journals and publications, and scientific papers have to be rigorously scrutinised by referees to check the ethics, logic and the statistics, before a paper can be approved for publication. A multitude of research papers worldwide fail to get published if they cannot meet the referees' standards.

If a paper is published, it means that clinical trials on large enough numbers of people have shown measurable benefits, but the most powerful evidence comes from 'meta-analysis', that is where all the known trials of a drug or treatment are put together mathematically. That way, relatively small effects and rare side-effects can be observed, as the largest numbers of people are involved.

Choosing the correct treatment in psychiatry can be difficult. There are a variety of approaches and drugs available, but no really clear pointers to which precise approach, or drug, will work in an individual. Good treatment in psychiatry takes account of the whole person, the personality, the circumstances and what view he or she has on life.

We are increasingly encouraged to use 'evidence-based' medicine in all areas of medicine – not just psychiatry. This involves using treatments that we know to work and have been shown to work in research. Good and sound though this approach is, there are limitations:

- In psychiatry we are often dealing with people over 65 years of age and relatively little research addresses them specifically.
- The 'best' treatment according to research may not be a practical or acceptable treatment to the person with

depression. A person, for very good reasons, may not be prepared to take a tablet, but may accept a syrup (there is not always a choice).

Electrical treatment may be the treatment of choice in some severe depressive illnesses. Some people will not accept this and alternatives (possibly less effective) have to be found. We know that cognitive behaviour therapy is very helpful in the treatment of depression. Sadly this may not be available either in general practice, or within the hospital setting, without a long wait. Evidence-based psychiatry is not nearly as clear-cut as, for example, the treatment of high blood pressure, where the person usually has less firmly held views on the choice of treatment. Negotiation of a treatment that is acceptable and helpful to the person is terribly important. Ultimately we still have to rely on our experience and acumen to make many judgements and decisions where there simply is not as yet cast-iron evidence.

How can I judge how my treatment is helping?

At first you are unlikely to notice a great deal. After a few days on antidepressants you may realise that your sleep is better in quality. Your moods may then become less labile; that means less variable. Irritability is reduced and, as your battery gradually recharges, you will find that you have more mental energy in reserve, and that you can cope better with life. Antidepressants are not stimulants or happy pills, so you don't start to feel happy, but your mood will gradually lift. This can take time. Don't give up too soon. A proper trial of medication may take as long as 2 months. If there is no change after this time, your doctor is likely to need to review things and reconsider your treatment.

As time goes by, taking an interest in your usual activities, hobbies, sports or pastimes will also help. You get stimulation and enjoyment from pleasurable activity again (that's why we call it 're-creation').

What books do doctors rely on for information about drugs?

We're all sent regular copies of the British National Formulary (the BNF). This contains information about every licensed drug in the UK. It is updated quarterly, and has information about drug costs, side-effects, and interactions. It disparages less effective remedies. It gives a thumbnail sketch of each licensed drug. Besides giving details of all medications used for depression, anxiety and other psychiatric conditions, it has good sections on prescribing in pregnancy, breastfeeding and childhood.

We are also sent a smaller monthly booklet called the *Monthly Index of Medical Specialities* (MIMS). If your doctor wants to check the dose of a drug, you will probably have seen the GP using one of these two booklets. Many of us now have all this information on our computer screens.

My GP has referred me to a psychiatrist. What will happen?

General practitioners refer only about 5% of people who are depressed to a specialist. Most people with depressive illness will be treated successfully and respond to treatment set up by their GP. If you are referred for an outpatient appointment, there is a high chance that you will need to attend only for a limited period. Two-thirds of people referred to psychiatric outpatient clinics will be helped in about four sessions. See also Chapter 7 which discusses hospital referral and treatment.

Antidepressant treatment for depression

General questions

How were antidepressants discovered?

The discovery of antidepressants was a lucky chance. The drug used for treating tuberculosis was found to brighten mood in depressed people, or they even became 'high'. This drug was developed into iproniazid, the first monoamine oxidase inhibitor.

At about the same time, another drug company was developing a preparation to help sedate and treat people with schizophrenia. They started working with an antihistamine-like drug and found it helped lift mood. This substance was developed into imipramine, the first widely used antidepressant. This family of drugs worked primarily on the noradrenaline system. Some years later, drugs that worked on serotonin (5-HT) systems were developed.

For about 40 years the choice of antidepressant was fairly limited, but then there was a very rapid expansion of new families of drugs.

How effective are these drugs?

The effects of active medication have always to be compared with the so-called placebo response – or the changes produced by an inert substance thought to be active by the person using it. About a third of depressed people will have a placebo response if given an inert tablet. They will feel better despite the fact that the substance has no known chemical effect. This effect happens in the treatment of a wide variety of illnesses from high blood pressure to epilepsy. It is not a reflection of the patient's intelligence, or general 'mind set', but rather a response of a normal human being to being given a substance that they believe is a treatment. Common placebo responses (whether an anti-depressant or any other tablet) are dry mouth, headache, nausea and drowsiness. All these 'side-effects' with a placebo are also found as side-effects of antidepressant medication. These same symptoms can also be symptoms of an untreated depressive illness. This makes evaluating side-effects, and the effects of illness more difficult.

What difference does drug treatment make?

Most depressive illness will get better given time, with or without treatment. However, drugs have a very important role in the treatment of depressive illness because they help reduce the unpleasantness of the illness, and speed up recovery. No anti-depressant is habit forming – this has been widely researched. About two-thirds of depressed people will improve given an anti-depressant, although they may not respond to the first drug they are given.

So when should antidepressants be prescribed?

The decision whether or not to prescribe an antidepressant depends on whether or not you are actually ill with depression (not merely low in mood). Having a 'reason' (or not) for being depressed, does not affect that decision. The signs of illness are biological, or consist of body changes that include:

- low mood with negative, and possibly suicidal, thoughts
- a change in sleep pattern
- a change in eating pattern (most often a loss of appetite)
- a change in activity level (either agitation or a slowing down of activity)
- a loss of sexual interest and performance, and
- poor concentration.

There are a variety of suggested mechanisms by which people become depressed (see Chapter 3).

How long do I need to go on taking an antidepressant?

This has been carefully researched and we tend to give longer courses of treatment now. If this is the first illness, you will need to take medication for a minimum of 6 months from the point at which you felt better (not from day one of taking the tablets). If this is a second episode, it is usually recommended that you have medication for 2–3 years. This may sound a very long time but, if you are feeling better, and are established on a tablet that you know and trust, it is a very good 'insurance policy' to staying well. If you are unfortunate enough to have had three or more episodes of depression in the past, it may be suggested that you take the medication for 5 years. Some elderly people who become very depressed may need to take medication for the rest of their lives.

If you do need to take medication for a relatively long period, try to regard it as a regular, necessary part of your daily routine, like an asthma sufferer using an inhaler.

I've been on antidepressants for 2 months but they haven't worked. My doctor says I might have treatment-resistant depression. What does this mean?

If a second course of antidepressants is given for an adequate time, and there is still no good response, the term 'treatment-resistant' depression is used. This does not mean that the illness cannot be treated, but it does mean that both doctor and patient have to keep working at finding a treatment strategy that works.

Treatment-resistant depression can be caused by:

- not taking the treatment prescribed
- stopping treatment too soon
- an accompanying physical illness, which has either caused the depression or is making it more difficult to treat
- alcohol abuse – drinking to try and feel better, which in fact makes mood worse
- unresolved family or social problems – depressive illness might well not respond to medication until the underlying problem is addressed.

There are *many* strategies available for treatment-resistant depression. You may be referred to the outpatient clinic for review. Try not to despair – it can be shifted.

Should I increase the dose? Would that help?

That depends on which drug you are taking. Most of the selective serotonin re-uptake inhibitors (SSRIs – see below) have a single dose suiting most people. The older tricyclic antidepressants (TCAs – see below) on the other hand have more leeway with dosage, and we can fine-tune this to suit the individual. Take careful advice from your GP before altering your dosage. Some psychiatrists use a combination of antidepressants, but this requires expert judgement to get it right.

My dad says 'Depressed people should just pull their socks up. They don't need drugs.' What can I say to him to put him straight?

Tell him that depression is an illness and can affect every area of our lives. The lack of drive and enthusiasm that goes with it can be pretty frustrating for family and friends, especially if their work or home responsibilities are being devolved to others, but it is just as much a medical condition, and just as disabling as, say, a broken leg. It might not look as though something is wrong, but there is.

The drugs we use are well proven, known to be effective and have prevented a great deal of human misery. Of course, self-help tactics are important too, but people may need to be prepared to use a variety of methods to get better. The drugs are not to be taken lightly either!

My gran is on antidepressants but I think she forgets her tablets She's on five tablets daily and it does seem complicated. What can we do?

Talk to your chemist about organising a 'dosette box'. This is a weekly calendar pack with spaces for the day's pills in morning, noon and night-time enclosures. The chemist can load this up for her weekly, and will arrange the necessary weekly prescriptions from her GP. All she has to do is open the compartment at mealtimes, and you can easily see if she has missed any. Some chemists can deliver these for the elderly, by arrangement. These boxes are also quite useful if she is going away on holiday.

I took an antidepressant for a few weeks but it didn't work. What should I do?

Probably you have not gone on for long enough. Antidepressants work slowly. You need to rebuild your levels of brain chemicals over a number of weeks and months. We believe you need to take an antidepressant for 8 weeks to give it a proper trial. You will probably see some improvement after 7–10 days. If there isn't any benefit, then your doctor may need to switch medication, or review the diagnosis. People who are drinking regularly are less likely to respond fully to antidepressants. A full course of treatment should last for 6 months after you get better, if it is the first time you have been treated.

Can I drink whilst taking antidepressants?

You can, but only in very modest amounts – say a glass of wine or half a pint of beer. Alcohol will exaggerate the sleepy effects of an antidepressant. *Never* have even the smallest amount of alcohol when you are on antidepressants and intend to drive. You will effectively become drunk much faster. Remember what happened to Princess Diana's chauffeur – and his passengers.

Can I drive while depressed or taking antidepressant medication?

This is a very difficult question. You certainly could drive whilst you are very depressed and many people knowingly or unknowingly do. There are no statutory regulations about this. In theory nobody who is taking antidepressants should drive. However, serious untreated depression can cause very poor driving because of lack of attention, slow reaction time and indecision. Someone who is not oversedated with medication and is feeling a lot stronger will be a much safer driver than an untreated depressed person. Some tablets, such as imipramine and similar drugs, cause drowsiness and slower reaction times even at a fairly low dose. The newer antidepressants are much less sedating. If somebody has to drive and needs medication, the latter would be the treatment of choice. If you are a driver of a heavy goods vehicle, you should not drive while taking anti-depressant medication.

Generally, if you feel well enough to drive, it is best to give yourself several practice runs in the car in a quiet road, in good light. Make sure that you would be safe if you had to do an emergency stop – if a child ran out into the road, for example. Do not embark on long motorway journeys. Recognise that you will tire faster than you would do normally, if you are depressed or on antidepressants. Be aware that your reaction times will be slower if you are on medication. Do not drink alcohol while on anti-depressants if you wish to drive (see question above).

Are there any antidepressant medications that haven't been tested on animals?

I'm afraid not. Every medication that doctors can prescribe has had to be extensively tested for safety, first in test-tubes, then in animals, then finally in human volunteers. Herbal remedies, which are not licensed as medications, are not checked for safety in this way. This does mean that their safety, effectiveness, correct dose and side-effects are less well understood. Some herbal remedies can be very effective, but can have lethal side-effects or interactions.

If you have a serious illness causing you distress, perhaps the wisest thing to do is to take the best established, most proven remedy.

Types of antidepressants

All the main groups of drugs are listed in Box 5.1.

Which antidepressant will suit me best?

There are now over 30 antidepressant drugs to choose from. However, new antidepressants are not more effective than older antidepressants – all antidepressants have the same efficacy. What varies between drugs are their side-effects particularly; secondly, the older antidepressants are much more dangerous if taken in overdose. Whichever antidepressant is used, significant improvement in mood is not usually seen for approximately 2 weeks.

Box 5.1 Medications commonly used for depression and anxiety

The manufacturers' trade names are included in brackets after the generic (chemical) names. Some drugs are not prescribable on the NHS; these are marked with an asterisk (*).

MAIN ANTIDEPRESSANTS

Tricyclic antidepressants (TCAs)
These drugs have been in use for the last 40 years. They are also helpful in phobic and obsessive-compulsive disorders (see Chapter 10). Some are more sedative than others, and this side-effect can help improve sleep patterns. They are contraindicated in pregnancy or if you have severe heart or liver disease, and caution is needed if you have prostate or urinary problems, or glaucoma.
Drugs include:

amitriptyline (Lentizol)	imipramine (Tofranil)
amoxapine (Asendis)	nortriptyline (Allegron)
clomipramine (Anafranil)	trimipramine(Surmontil)
dothiepin (Prothiaden)	
doxepin (Sinequan)	

Newer drugs include:
    lofepramine (Gamanil)

Selective serotonin re-uptake inhibitors (SSRIs)
These are less sedative than TCAs, and have different side-effects. They can cause nausea and increased symptoms of anxiety initially.
Drugs include:

citalopram (Cipramil)	paroxetine (Seroxat)
fluoxetine (Prozac)	sertraline (Lustral)
fluvoxamine (Faverin)	

Monoamine oxidase inhibitors (MAOIs)
These were the first antidepressants to be developed, and are still potent and effective. They must be used with caution because of interactions with many other drugs and foods, in particular those rich in the amino acid tyramine. Foods to avoid include: cheese, Bovril, Oxo, broad bean pods, banana skins, yeast extracts including Marmite, pickled foods, textured vegetable protein, dark beers, chianti wines, low alcohol drinks, and food that isn't fresh!
Drugs include:
    phenelzine (Nardil)
    tranylcypromine(Parnate)
    moclobemide(Manerix) – a recently developed 'reversible' MAOI is much easier to use with far lower risk of dangerous drug interactions.

Selective noradrenaline re-uptake inhibitors (NARIs)
These have been developed to try and reduce the above side-effects.
reboxetine (Edronax) is in this group.

Noradrenaline and selective serotonin antidepressants (NASSAs)
Another highly selective class of drug, these are useful if anxiety, sleep
disturbance, nausea or sexual problems occur with other medication.
mirtazapine (Zispin) is in this group.

5-hydroxytryptamine (5-HT) antagonists
These are helpful if sleep disturbance and sexual difficulty occur with other
drugs.
nefazodone (Dutonin) is in this group.

Other
venlafaxine (Efexor XL) has effects on both 5-HT and NARI systems.
maprotiline (Ludiomil) is a tetracyclic.

TRANQUILLISERS

Tranquillisers or calming drugs can cause sedation, drowsiness, impaired
dexterity and reaction times. There will be warnings on the label about driving or
operating machinery. Avoid mixing alcohol with any tranquilliser.

Minor tranquillisers
Benzodiazepines
These are also used as sleeping tablets.
Good points: Few side-effects, and safe in overdosage.
Bad points: Longer acting ones can cause drowsiness the next day. May cause
unsteadiness or falls in the elderly. Habit forming; should **not** be used for longer
than 2 weeks, and preferably intermittently.
Drugs include:

bromazepam (Lexotan)*	loprazolam
chlordiazepoxide (Librium)	lorazepam (Ativan)
clobazam (Frisium)*	lormetazepam
clorazepate (Tranxene)*	nitrazepam (Mogadon)
diazepam (Valium)	oxazepam*
flunitrazepam (Rohypnol)*	temazepam
flurazepam (Dalmane)*	

Other
buspirone (Buspar)

Notes on sleeping tablets: We regard sleeping tablets as helpful for a crisis,
but in general longer term use is to be avoided. There is no ideal sleeping tablet.
All of these can be dangerous if misused – and some are lethal.

Box 5.1 Medications commonly used for depression (continued)

Some others
    chloral hydrate (Welldorm)   zolpidem (Stilnoct)
    chlormethiazole (Heminevrin)   zopiclone (Zimovane)
    zaleplon (Sonata)

Antihistamines. Also used for allergies, they are mildly sedating. Some can be bought over the counter.
Drugs include:
    hydroxyzine (Atarax, Ucerax)
    promethazine (Phenergan)

Major tranquillisers
These are often used for treating psychotic illness. They can be helpful in treating anxiety symptoms associated with depression, particularly in lower doses. In higher doses they can cause 'extrapyramidal' side-effects (muscular stiffness, tremor and odd movements) but they are non-addictive.
Drugs include:
    chlorpromazine (Largactil)
    droperidol (Droleptan)
    flupenthixol (Depixol, Fluanxol)
    haloperidol (Haldol, Serenace, Dozic)
    perphenazine (Fentazin)
    trifluoperazine (Stelazine)

Barbiturates
These potent drugs are seldom used outside hospital in view of their potential for addiction, abuse, and severe withdrawal. Lethal in overdose or with alcohol, they also affect how you break down other drugs in the liver. They are all Controlled Drugs under the Misuse of Drugs regulations.
Drugs include:
    amylobarbitone (Amytal, Sodium Amytal)
    butobarbitone (Soneryl)
    quinalbarbitone (Seconal, Tuinal)

Mood stabilisers
Lithium. Used to treat bipolar disorder (manic depression) and unipolar depression. It helps stabilise mood; it can be used in treatment-resistant depression. It can also be used to help prevent relapse of mood disorder. Regular monitoring of blood levels, and thyroid and kidney function is needed.
Other drugs that can also be used as mood stabilisers:
    carbamazepine (Tegretol)
    sodium valproate (Epilim)

TCAs (tricyclic antidepressants)

TCAs are still very useful drugs. They are good at reducing anxiety (and work quickly in this respect). They are also helpful in re-establishing sleep. In addition they have some painkilling action and, if depression is associated with pain, they can be very useful. If you have had a previous episode of depression, and responded well to a tricyclic, it is likely to be a first choice of drug again. What has worked in the past, is highly likely to work now.

However, there are disadvantages. They are potentially lethal in overdose. They can oversedate you and slow down your reaction time. This effect causes potential hazards when you are driving or operating machinery. They cannot be taken by people who suffer from heart disease or have a particular type of glaucoma (raised pressure within the eye).

Common side-effects of TCAs are dry mouth, constipation, difficulty in emptying the bladder, blurred vision and dizziness on a sudden change of posture (postural hypotension). They can contribute to weight gain. You might not get any of these side-effects or you could get several. If the depression is helped, the experience of one or two of these side-effects in moderate degree is almost always an acceptable alternative to depressive illness.

Quite commonly people adjust to their antidepressant – a side-effect that was troublesome at the onset of treatment may fade within 1 or 2 weeks.

SSRIs (selective serotonin re-uptake inhibitors)

These are newer drugs than tricyclics. They are not more effective – they are equally effective as the older drugs. SSRIs are not potentially lethal in overdose, which is obviously important when someone has had suicidal thoughts. The SSRIs have a different range of side-effects from the tricyclics, and these include:

- gastric upset, nausea and decreased appetite
- diarrhoea
- sleep disturbance (this may be transient or continuing)
- sexual difficulty (unfortunately, this side-effect can persist through treatment and may be a reason for some to stop the medication)

- headache (this usually stops after the first week of treatment)
- excessive sweating
- increased anxiety levels (initially only – later they decrease anxiety).

Sometimes a short course of a drug like diazepam (Valium) is given to make the onset of treatment more manageable. The diazepam is then stopped.

What happens when you stop an SSRI?

SSRIs, like all other antidepressants, are non-addictive, but a discontinuation syndrome can occur when an SSRI is stopped suddenly. This is more likely to happen with the SSRIs that have a short 'half-life', i.e. they are eliminated from the body in a relatively short time. SSRIs which 'last' longer are much less likely to do this, e.g. fluoxetine (Prozac). Discontinuation syndrome can cause dizziness or a feeling of imbalance, tingling in the hands and feet, 'flu-like symptoms and anxiety. Only about one in five people taking these drugs experience it (and very often to an extremely mild degree). It *can* happen after missing just one dose of the medication. In order to try and avoid this, keep a spare tablet in your wallet or purse so that, if you forget your morning dose, you can take it later at work or whilst out. Although the discontinuation syndrome is unpleasant, it does not cause any long-term difficulties and rarely poses a big problem.

Prozac

Does Prozac make you aggressive? I know someone who became violent after starting an antidepressant.

Prozac is one of the SSRIs and they all work in the same way by improving serotonin levels in the brain. There is no hard evidence that any SSRI will make you aggressive. Prozac has a stimulant side-effect profile. Whilst this is not strong, it is noticeable. This side-effect can be beneficial – someone who is quite flat and low may feel more alert and stimulated early on in treatment, but this is quite different from the antidepressant effects.

Some people describe the stimulation rather like the effect of a cup of coffee, i.e. pleasantly alerting. This is not likely to make you behave out of character. Did the person you describe have any previous history of aggressive behaviour? If he is quite highly strung or keyed up, e.g. an 'angry young man', he may have been better on a neutral or mildly sedative antidepressant.

Lithium

I have bipolar disorder, and have had several spells of elated mood; once I had to stay in hospital. Can I do anything to stop these happening?

Long-term mood stabilising medication can help prevent your moods swinging up and down so drastically. Prophylaxis (meaning preventative treatment) is usually recommended if your moods are persistently unstable, for example if you have had more than one mood swing in 2 years.

Several drugs are used for this; lithium is the best known. It has no direct action as a tranquilliser but stabilises brain chemistry. Other drugs are also used: carbamazepine (Tegretol) and sodium valproate (Epilim), used in the treatment of epilepsy, are also effective as mood stabilisers. Carbamazepine can interfere with the action of the oral contraceptive pill. This will need to be discussed with your doctor. There are also some other drug interactions. Ask your pharmacist if in doubt.

Once you start a mood stabiliser, you will probably need it for a minimum of 3 years. There is some evidence that, if you stop lithium before the 3 years are up, the rate of relapse can increase. A few people need to stay on a mood stabiliser permanently.

I'm on lithium for recurrent mood swings. My doctor says I need blood tests. Why is this?

Lithium is a natural substance and is in the same chemical family as the salt we put on food. Lithium will have little or no therapeutic effect if the level in the bloodstream is too low. If the level is too high, then toxic side-effects occur.

For the lithium to be used safely and usefully, a certain blood level of the drug needs to be reached. When you first start lithium, the level of the drug is tested about 5 days later to check that the level is satisfactory. The level of lithium is tested 12 hours after the last dose of lithium. This will give the average blood level over 24 hours. A few minutes either way is fine, but not an hour or so. The drug dose may need to be raised or lowered, or left the same, depending on the result. Once you are established on lithium, its dose remains fairly settled, and checks need then be done only once every 3 months. If you have a severe gut upset with diarrhoea and vomiting, or you become markedly dehydrated for any other reason, lithium will become more concentrated in the blood, until things correct themselves. Too much sunbathing on a very hot beach or a hangover, for example, can make you dehydrated. If you are unable to keep fluids down, leave off the lithium that day and get in touch with your doctor or nurse. Try to get your fluids back to normal levels as soon as possible.

If you do start on lithium treatment, your chemist will give you an information sheet about its safe use. Toxic side-effects of lithium treatment, i.e. changes seen when the drug level is too high, include a tremor (but this can also occur when the levels are absolutely normal), drowsiness, confusion, giddiness and slurring of speech.

Lithium can transform people's lives – but it is a drug that needs to be respected.

Once a year, blood tests are taken to check kidney function and thyroid gland function. If the kidneys are not working to capacity, lithium levels can become raised into the toxic level. Lithium is got rid of by the kidneys. After fairly long-term use of lithium, the thyroid gland can slow down. The thyroid gland (in the neck) regulates body metabolism. If the thyroid slows down, we slow down and can put on weight; mood can also be affected and thoughts can become sluggish.

Safety of antidepressants

My husband is in recovery from alcoholism. Is it safe for him to be treated with psychiatric drugs?

In most cases, yes it is. Once he is well clear of the alcohol problem, most antidepressants are quite safe and are not addictive. Most psychiatric drugs cannot be abused. The big exception to this rule would be the so-called minor tranquillisers: the benzodiazepines (diazepam, chlordiazepoxide, lorazepam, temazepam, etc.). These certainly *do* have abuse potential.

Remember your husband is vulnerable to any addictive substance, not just alcohol, and these medications could be risky for him unless they are carefully controlled.

If he is a member of AA, read the pamphlet *The AA member – medications & other drugs* (see Appendix 2). AA philosophy calls tranquillisers 'dry drinks' and members of AA groups are often strongly against any sort of medication that alters how you perceive reality, in particular the tranquillisers.

Sadly, some well-meaning members of AA groups, trying to avoid unnecessary medication, have talked other members out of having their depression treated with antidepressants, and some ill people have killed themselves as a result. AA's *official* attitude toward medication is definitely that it is necessary for certain illnesses including depression.

My previous doctor used to give me Valium when I went to see him about stress and depression, but the new one will not. Why is she so reluctant?

Minor tranquillisers (mainly the family of drugs called benzo-diazepines) certainly were used too much. When they came out in the 1960s, they were so much safer than the older drugs for calming people, such as the barbiturates, that they were overprescribed. Their addictive potential was not recognised initially. Now we know better. Whilst they do calm you down and help you get off to sleep, they will not help depression itself. They have no antidepressant effect.

However, a short course of these drugs during a crisis can be very useful; of course, self-help and friendly support is the best drug, but sometimes you cannot just switch off and get a good night's sleep when you're stressed and low. If sleeping tablets are prescribed, it is best to try and limit them for use over a number of days, rather than weeks: 3 days' treatment may well be enough to break the pattern of bad sleep or tension. Some people sleep better if they know they have a small supply of sleeping tablets to eke out, even if they scarcely use them.

Your doctor isn't alone in trying to minimise the use of these drugs. They have an excellent safety record but have certainly been overprescribed. They are not a treatment for depression.

I was taking Valium for years, and have had real trouble stopping it. My GP says I actually have an underlying depression, and has started me on an antidepressant, which seems to help. I now attend a Tranquilliser Users' Support Group, which gives me good support, but they are very against people taking antidepressants, and tell me I should stop them. Who is right?

Well-meaning organisations such as some of the alcohol and tranquilliser self-help bodies do sometimes have this attitude. Although they have the best of intentions, and are generally trying to help people to live their lives without what they see as the crutch of medication, they are wrong.

In our experience, many people who have in the past been prescribed tranquillisers such as Valium on a long-term basis do actually have symptoms of underlying depression, or other conditions such as social phobia or agoraphobia, which will be helped by proper, full courses of standard antidepressants. Stopping antidepressants part of the way through a course may actually make the condition more difficult to treat subsequently, and some people come to harm in this way.

So although the work of groups such as these is very supportive, do not let anyone tell you that you should not be taking your antidepressants, or that they are addictive.

Side-effects

Will I get side-effects?

All medication causes side-effects. The quest is to find an anti-depressant that is effective and tolerable. The same medication may not work for one person, but works brilliantly for another. You cannot tell before you start treatment which tablet is best suited to which person.

Always take the medication as advised. If you have any queries, do ask the doctor or pharmacist. Pharmacists are quite rightly proud of the service they offer, explaining queries about medication. It is a very important part of their work.

What happens if the tablets don't agree with me?

If you cannot get on with your treatment, do say. Always tell the doctor if you have stopped taking the tablets or are worried. We know that a large number of people, possibly as many as 50%, will discontinue their medication over the course of 6 months. About a quarter of people who stop medication do so because of unpleasant side-effects. Within the range of antidepressants, the overall rate of dropout because of side-effects of medication is a little greater with the older tricyclic drugs compared with the newer SSRIs. The differences are not large.

Very often side-effects of medication are transient, and will decrease if you persevere with the drug. Some people will need what looks like a high dose of medication, others are lucky enough to respond to less. Each person responds to drugs in an individual and slightly different manner.

Are people more likely to harm themselves when they start antidepressants?

Antidepressants do not cause people to harm themselves and, on the contrary, save many lives by preventing depression getting to the stage where suicide is contemplated. Someone who is severely depressed to the point of wishing to harm themselves may, however, act on this feeling when an antidepressant starts to work, simply because they start to get a little more drive and get the energy to put their plans into action. Someone who is this unwell should be under close specialist care, perhaps in hospital. If a friend or relative is this low, and talking about self-harm, tell their doctor. See the section on *Self-harm* in Chapter 9 for more information.

Will an antidepressant make me feel high or stimulated? I don't like to think that I might feel out of control.

Almost always the answer is no.

Antidepressants are not mood-altering drugs, like Ecstasy and amphetamines are. If somebody who is not depressed is given an antidepressant, their mood will not change. Moods will only be shifted by antidepressants if you are depressed – the shift will be from low to normal mood.

However, if you have a predisposition to elated mood swings as part of a manic-depressive illness, several antidepressant drugs can cause 'high' mood. This is unusual, but can pose a serious problem.

How can I get rid of the side-effects of my antidepressant medication?

You may be noticing dry mouth or constipation if you are on a tricyclic, and indigestion or nausea if you are taking an SSRI.

You are likely to develop tolerance to these symptoms as time passes, so be patient. If nausea is a problem, it may be helpful if you start your SSRI at half dose until you get used to it. A dry mouth can be helped by chewing gum. Some constipation –

usually mild – is quite a common side effect with antidepressants. Prevention is the best remedy: drink 2–3 pints of fluid daily, and take plenty of fruit and fibre in your diet. Lactulose is one of the milder laxatives sometimes prescribed for this symptom, and is also available over the counter from a chemist.

Addiction to treatment

Are antidepressants addictive?

No. This is a question that has been widely researched over very many years. There is no evidence that any antidepressant drug is addictive (or habit forming). However, it does need to be said that some antidepressants are more difficult to decrease and stop than others. The older tricyclic antidepressants, are relatively easy to decrease and stop, whereas some of the newer anti-depressants, particularly paroxetine (Seroxat), can sometimes cause symptoms initially when the dose is decreased and stopped.

This phenomenon is called a 'discontinuation syndrome' and is like the symptoms that prompted the doctor to start the medication in the first place, such as anxiety, tingling in the hands or feet, and a feeling of being 'spaced out'. Over half the general population wrongly believe that antidepressants are addictive. This is the major reason for people giving up medication too soon.

I had a problem with substance abuse and I have to be really careful about what I take. Will I get addicted to antidepressants?

No. Antidepressants are definitely not addictive substances. Many people who have been through a recovery and rehabilitation programme for addictions have quite rightly been carefully trained to avoid mood-altering substances. They are encouraged to learn to live in the real world, however uncomfortable it may be, rather than blotting it out or escaping from it. Alcohol, tranquillisers and stimulants (whether legal or illegal ones) obviously come into this category. However, antidepressants do not alter your sensory perceptions. They do not make you feel high, happy or excited. They do not prevent you from perceiving what's happening all around you in real life or help you escape from it. So you will not – repeat not – get addicted to them.

You mention that drugs like Valium are addictive. Does this apply to everybody?

Valium and the rest of its family, the benzodiazepines, are certainly effective at reducing anxiety. However, current prescribing guidelines are very clear that these drugs should only be used for a maximum of 2–4 weeks, and only for severe, disabling, distressing anxiety. Habituation (addiction) can all too easily occur if they are used for longer periods. This means that the effect wears off and you have to increase the dose to get the same effect. Stopping these drugs after a longer period of time can also be difficult and lead to withdrawal symptoms. These drugs can have a disinhibiting effect, and paradoxically make you excited or even aggressive, by reducing your normal self-control mechanisms.

The same drugs are commonly used as sleeping tablets, and again we do advise that they are best used only in short spells, for a few days at a time is best. Longer use can lead to rebound insomnia, where your sleep becomes worse when you stop the drug.

Having made that general caution about these drugs, it is true that some people are more vulnerable to addictions than others. We do talk about 'addictive personalities', people who are particularly vulnerable to becoming addicted, and this can take the form of addiction to alcohol, nicotine, prescribed or street drugs, or to comforting, exciting or risky behaviours, such as overeating, computer games, gambling – and even sex. It seems clear that these behaviours may run in families, and that genetics play a part in addictions of all kinds.

If someone has had a problem with alcohol or other drugs in the past, doctors need to be particularly cautious when prescribing anything that alters mood. However, antidepressants and the major tranquillisers (chlorpromazine, haloperidol and the new major tranquillisers, like olanzepine) are not addictive.

How can I avoid discontinuation symptoms? I've been on an SSRI for 9 months and I want to stop it soon.

Tail off your medications gradually over a month. Some people don't notice any problem at all, others are more perceptive to these symptoms. You can get some antidepressants in liquid form if you want to subdivide the final dose into smaller and smaller amounts. Usually just taking one dose on alternate days does the trick.

Other forms of therapy

Psychotherapy (counselling)

What is psychotherapy?

It is 'talking treatment' or, more precisely, as Dr Anthony Storr defined, it is 'the art of alleviating personal difficulties through the agency of words and a personal, professional relationship'. The professional relationship is established with the object of removing, or modifying, existing symptoms, disturbed ways of behaving, and helping to bring about a positive development in your personality and social life. It leads to an understanding and acceptance of ourselves. The treatment takes place in a safe setting at a time and location set aside for it, with an expectation of confidentiality.

What types are there?

The range of psychotherapeutic methods is enormous.

The most common form of psychotherapy is *informal psychotherapy or counselling*. This can be offered by professional people, but is much more commonly encountered in everyday life in our routine contact with people. It is what happens in the course of normal caring social interaction. It is the help that people give each other when they are trying to help a friend or colleague. It involves giving support and listening, but not expecting any kind of change – just being there for someone.

The next division within psychotherapy, is *formal psychotherapy or counselling*. This takes place in a particular setting at a time that is set aside with a person who has a qualification to help. The psychotherapy may be supportive, or it may be dynamic psychotherapy.

In *supportive (formal) psychotherapy*, the most common type of psychotherapy, the therapist is aiming to restore the person to their previous level of functioning or, sometimes, just maintain the status quo. Great changes are not the goal. The role of the therapist is as a listener, albeit an 'active listener'. The aim is to try and reduce the problem into a manageable proportion, to reflect back what has been said in order to clarify the situation, and hopefully to make it easier to see a way forward.

Dynamic psychotherapy is perhaps more challenging. During treatment the therapist is aiming to bring about a change – possibly a permanent change – in the way someone is dealing with their difficulties. A very wide range of techniques are used in this form of treatment.

Questions about psychotherapy

What is the difference between counselling and psychotherapy?

The distinction is often very fine. Generally, a psychotherapist would have had longer, and more formal, training than people who work as counsellors.

What should I expect during psychotherapy or counselling?

Expect to work hard. Therapy is not a passive exercise. You are not going to be told what to do – you will not be told to leave your wife, quit your job, sell your house or change your life. What

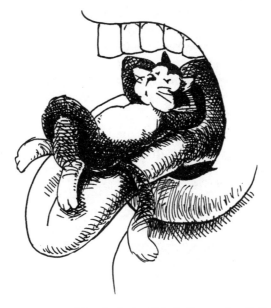

you will be encouraged to do is to think through all the possibilities of solutions and changes that are available to you, and to see what is likely to be best for you. The therapist will act as a sort of catalyst, enabling things to happen a little faster. Good therapists use 'active listening' techniques that help you put whatever is going on in your mind into a clearer form. Once you have started defining your feelings – hearing yourself explaining and telling someone else what the problem is – this often in turn 'explains' it to you too. If you are told by someone what to do, you will not 'own' that solution nor will you feel committed to it. You will not feel energised to make the solution work for you. If the decision is 'wrong', it can be dismissed as someone else's idea rather than potentially a situation that can be turned around and used to good benefit.

Psychotherapy is aimed at enabling someone to make up their own mind about their own lives. We have much more power over our lives than we tend to realise, and there is nobody who knows as much about us as ourselves. You are an expert on you.

Therapy is challenging. You need to feel fairly strong in order to deal with things honestly. You will not be able to cope well with talking therapies if you are clinically depressed. You may well need treatment with medication before embarking on therapy. It is a good rule to see a doctor before starting treatment.

One of the best ways that a GP can help prepare someone for successful counselling and psychotherapy is by treating clinical depression first. Your GP is a good source of information on how to get access to counselling.

Is psychotherapy always done on a one-to-one basis?

No. Some very powerful psychotherapy is done with people working as couples, families or in groups – *group therapy*. There are also some specialised *support groups* in which help is given, and mutual support gained by people who share the same problem, for example agoraphobia, overeating or diabetes. Group therapy will also include very widespread and successful groups like AA and NA. The setting, the style and format of these support groups will vary widely.

What therapies are available on the NHS or voluntary sector?

What is available in the NHS does vary depending very much on local resources. Within a hospital district, there should be a psychotherapy service led by a consultant psychotherapist, who would have junior doctors and a team of other professionals working alongside. The NHS psychotherapy services have to be highly selective. It is, sadly, a scarce resource, and waiting times can be lengthy.

Outside NHS hospitals, there is a wide range from traditional and well-established psychoanalytical psychotherapy, to counselling sessions that go on in GP surgeries. There are many private sources of psychotherapy or counselling , and a number of charities also provide a good service. Your GP will be able to advise on reputable local resources. A considerable number of people receiving psychotherapy have been referred by their GPs, although many will refer themselves directly to a psychotherapist or counsellor.

How can I choose a good private psychotherapist?

There are some very good psychotherapists available, but there are also, of course, some quacks. One of the safest ways of ensuring that you are having treatment with a properly trained therapist is to check that they are on the United Kingdom Counsel for Psychotherapy (UKCP) Register. Before approaching a private psychotherapist, do make enquiries. A good therapist will not mind this at all. Ask what kind of treatment you are going to be offered and try to arrange to have a preliminary meeting to discuss what the therapist has on offer and what you feel you could get out of therapy. It will also be important to discuss the time that may be involved in treatment. Some therapists are very skilled at brief intervention, other therapists will want to spend many more sessions with their patients. Short therapy is not necessarily bad therapy, and long therapy is not necessarily good therapy.

What might private psychotherapy cost?

Costs will be higher in London. An experienced well-qualified psychotherapist would charge anything from about £35 to £80, or perhaps even £100, an hour. Paying more does not necessarily mean that you are getting better therapy. Therapists in training, who are being supervised, charge less than a therapist who is fully trained. Remember that, if someone is charging a very low fee over a long course of time, you may in fact spend more money than if you were having a shorter course of therapy being charged at average rates.

I have been attending counselling and after the third session I was very upset. The counsellor seemed to be tough with me when I was already feeling bad. Is this fair?

If you are dealing with a difficult problem, it is likely that you are going to have to examine feelings and behaviour honestly. Sometimes reality is harsh, and you will not be helped by somebody avoiding difficult and painful topics. Almost always, if there is going to be a major change, a great deal of effort has to be spent – 'no gain without pain'. Confrontation may well be necessary during this process. A good counsellor will know how to achieve this in a controlled, respectful and safe way. If you do find anything within a therapy session difficult, this needs to be discussed. Looking at the reason why something is difficult, and finding a new way of handling it *could* be very fruitful.

My family want me to see a counsellor, but I am not sure that I am strong enough at present to start talking about difficult things.

This is a very important point. Dynamic psychotherapy with somebody who is clinically depressed is very likely to be totally unproductive. If you are experiencing very low mood, supportive talking or therapy will be helpful and sustaining. Some people will need medication initially and then, when they are less depressed, they can make good use of talking treatments. The opposite is sometimes true – some people need to talk things through extensively before they realise that they are actually ill. The process by which they have become ill with depression could have been slow and insidious. There may be a resistance to accepting that illness is present. It may not be apparent until the person has had an opportunity to reflect on the fact that their decision-making, their prevailing mood, their sleep, appetite and libido may all have changed and could be linked to illness that medication could help.

What sort of things will a therapist do with me?

A good therapist will enable you to feel settled and safe enough to talk openly about how you are feeling. An early part of that process, during which trust is developed, is that a therapist will listen in an empathising and understanding way. Therapists need to be totally non-condemnatory, accepting what they hear. They, through the act of their listening, will give the message that what they are hearing is neither shocking, anger making or shaming. Unconditional acceptance of what is being said, without judgement, is very necessary.

The relationship that develops between a psychotherapist and the patient is very special and safe. Dependence on the therapist can become a problem. It is important that both patient and therapist are aware of this. A good therapist will not be frightened by somebody being very moody at times during their treatment, if they feel that they are leading the patient to a point where they will be stronger and more independent. Good therapy has a clear beginning, middle, and a well-timed and well-planned ending.

My daughter has been going to a counsellor for 2 years and doesn't seem able to make up her mind about anything without first asking her counsellor.

There are undoubtedly some counsellors and therapists who are not aware enough of the risk of dependence – and perhaps even sometimes foster dependence. Good psychotherapy or counselling will enable someone to make decisions. A counselling session can be very usefully used to weigh up the pros and cons of a situation. Using the time to discuss a difficulty is very different from expecting to be told what to do.

Does counselling help prevent post-traumatic stress disorder (PTSD)? We deal with the public in a difficult part of town. Staff do get verbally abused at our front desk sometimes, and this can be quite shocking. Some staff have gone off sick after incidents. Shouldn't our employer be obliged to provide counselling?

You would imagine the answer would be a resounding yes. Whenever there's a major disaster we hear of 'teams of counsellors' being brought in. However, there is no real evidence from a number of trials that have been done on this question showing that a one-off debriefing session reduces psychological distress, anxiety, depression, or other psychological symptoms, or prevents PTSD occurring. The conclusion from the trials was that compulsory debriefing of victims of trauma should cease.

On reflection, perhaps, this is not surprising. We all deal with shocks and upsets in our own ways. Verbal or physical violence does invade the very core of our own privacy, and trying to intervene in someone's private feelings at a time of upset might add to the unwelcome invasion of the 'self', however well meant it is. Maybe it's not helpful to review at length and rehearse what happened to you; might this fix it in your mind rather than help you get through it?

Friendly support and sympathy and the offer of time out – if wanted – to get over the upset may be the best approach, rather than a more official exploration of someone's wounded feelings, which may be intrusive, even disruptive.

Some staff may want to carry on as normal after a shock, others will need to let off steam, then or later. It is so important to support colleagues who have had an unpleasant experience. Tea and sympathy always help, but the evidence is clear that obligatory counselling (which may be a contradictory term anyway – you can't compel someone to confide in you) doesn't help, and could in fact make the situation worse.

What therapy works best?

Without a doubt, cognitive behaviour therapy (see below) is the best researched psychotherapy. This is almost certainly because it is much more easily measurable than other sorts of therapy. Cognitive behaviour therapy tends to focus on one or two symptoms and so outcomes are much more easily measured.

In psychotherapy in general, the recovery rate after treatment is about 65% – roughly two-thirds of people improve with psychotherapy. Time does heal. There is a spontaneous recovery rate of about 48% over time. Good psychotherapy can undoubtedly speed up the process. Even if an illness does appear to be slow to respond, good psychotherapy is extremely likely to enable someone to use all the resources that they have, and function better.

Can psychotherapy in depression ever be harmful?

Yes, occasionally it can. About 5% of people treated with psychotherapy do become worse. This is not a reflection of the calibre

of their therapist but indicates that some people will 'decompen-
sate', causing them to function less well. Psychotherapy is hard
work and challenging. If you are very fragile, there may not be
enough mental energy to take on the treatment. Timing is all
important.

Is counselling overrated?

Perhaps you are suggesting that people refer to counselling as a
solution for everything nowadays. Certainly it is often mentioned
as an almost knee-jerk response to many sorts of crisis. Perhaps
we can reflect that, in the 'good old days', our society was less
mobile, with stronger family ties, greater job security, and a more
settled social order. Did the Church, the Squire, the Boss and the
Family supply the support and stability then, that we are
nowadays trying to replace with trained counsellors via schools,
workplaces and the health service?

We now have material benefits, a life expectancy, and a
standard of living in this country that our grandparents would
never have dreamed of. Is there a greater level of stress and
strain, and less domestic, religious, and marital stability
nowadays, to go with these undoubted material benefits, or are
we less likely to put up with unhappiness, more likely to
reasonably expect good health and our share of well-being?

I think I'd prefer to start counselling before I consider taking medication, but my doctor suggests otherwise. Who is right?

It's good to talk; however, some people who are significantly
depressed definitely need to start medication before they can
embark on looking at their lives in detail. Considering difficult
things that have happened can be very traumatic. If your moods
are up and down, and you're not sleeping properly, the last thing
you need to be dealing with is tough issues from the past.

Some people may actually be put at greater risk of self-harm by
being given insights (or perhaps developing false ones) into
themselves before they are mentally strong enough to deal with

them. Using the medication first, to give people more coping resources before engaging in counselling, can be very helpful. Sometimes people seem to make little progress with counselling, perhaps because they're too depressed to benefit from it properly.

I've been seeing a counsellor for 2 years about my depression but I just feel worse. What should I do?

This can happen. If you've got the major symptoms of depressive illness despite counselling you should think very carefully about going onto some medication. Some people need to talk before they are ready to start treatment, others need to take medication to help them become ready to talk about things. If your sleep is dreadful and your concentration is shot, you aren't going to do yourself much justice with your counsellor. Another thing that may delay progress is using alcohol or street drugs to try and control symptoms.

Perhaps, too, you should re-evaluate your counselling. Is it goal-orientated, or open-ended? It is difficult to see the wood for the trees sometimes. Some sorts of counselling are very focused with agreed goals and targets, and limited to an agreed number of sessions.

Sometimes counsellors and their clients can get into rather a cosy rut together and, with the best will in the world, important or uncomfortable changes just don't get made. Counselling should be more than just support – it should lead to change being enabled.

In a minority of people, difficulties are very deep-seated and then long-term work with a counsellor or therapist may help.

What evidence is there that counselling helps?

Some general practices – not all – are fortunate enough to have counsellors attached to them. Other GPs may have made good links with local voluntary or private counsellors. All this costs money. Can we justify using Health Service resources on counselling, and do people who are paying for this sort of service receive worthwhile benefit for their money?

Counselling has to justify itself, like any other service. The results of early research projects were rather ambiguous, but a recent large systematic review looked stringently at the benefits of counsellors trained to British Association of Counsellors and Psychotherapists (BACP) standards, working in general practices. Results were mildly encouraging. They found 'a modest but significant improvement in symptom levels' and 'high levels of patient satisfaction' among people who received counselling. People like counselling, but it may not be as potent a treatment as we would like.

This evidence is welcome because it gives us good ammunition to get better resources for counselling in General Practice. At present there are staff shortages, a variable level of provision of counselling depending on where you are, and long waiting lists. We need to improve this.

Psychotherapy can, as we have seen, provide a non-directive and non-judgmental setting in which to work at your difficulties. The therapist will attempt to help explain what has happened and perhaps trace the origins of your style of coping. It will engender hope, and help kindle a feeling of mastery over problems.

Other therapies address *specific problems*. These therapies are behaviour therapy, cognitive behaviour therapy, and inter-personal therapy. The therapist in this situation focuses on addressing particular problems, and they have a specific aim in treatment – there is a very clear end point.

Behaviour therapy

The techniques of behaviour therapy are based on 'learning theory' – from the knowledge we have about how patterns of behaviour are learnt (and therefore changed). The aim of treatment is to change a *behaviour* rather than thoughts and feelings. It does not look at the genesis of the problem. The aim of treatment is to decrease symptoms.

The symptoms are viewed as unhelpful, difficult behaviours that have arisen because of faulty learning. The aim is to replace these with more appropriate and healthy behaviour. This can be very frightening. In a phobic person, for example, you cannot expect someone with a spider phobia to be comfortable with a spider crawling on their hand in the first treatment session – gradual gaining of experience, and careful timing is all important.

Behaviour therapy is a very powerful treatment for specific phobias, such as spiders or open spaces (see Chapter 10). It is also very useful in the treatment of obsessional compulsive disorder (see Chapter 10).

Cognitive behaviour therapy

This therapy came about as a development from behaviour therapy. 'Maladaptive' or unhelpful behaviour or feelings can be strongly reinforced and heightened by our thinking patterns. If you are depressed, the situation can be made much worse by negative thinking. This negative thinking is not just a symptom of depression but one of the most important agents in perpetuating the illness. Depressed people can frequently misinterpret what is said and what happens in the environment around them. What was mildly negative rapidly becomes intolerably gloomy. Self-esteem and expectations of oneself plummet. If the triggers to negative thinking can be identified, and challenged by the therapist, the assumptions made are examined and challenged to good effect. It is a clear and orderly form of treatment, and very persuasive.

A lot of the negative and bad thinking that we see in depressive illness isn't just a symptom of depression but one of the most important things that keeps it going. It's a vicious circle. People get lower and lower, and feel worse and worse about themselves. The aim of cognitive behaviour therapy is to challenge those negative thoughts, to get the patient to gradually decrease them, by questioning them, and questioning the underlying assumptions that led to those thoughts.

This involves recording automatic bad thoughts and keeping a 'thoughts diary' of them, and seeing how they challenge those negative thoughts. Then we encourage the person to try out other ways, rather than being stuck with their automatic thoughts and behaviour. Automatic thoughts can be very destructive. Some examples might be:

- If you've woken up feeling bad one morning, then the whole day's going to be bad.
- Just because a passer-by avoids making eye contact with you, you're ugly.
- Just because somebody didn't stop and talk to you at length in the morning coffee break, they don't like you – therefore nobody likes you at work, and therefore everything you do, every part of your life, is useless.

We then teach people to do 'reality testing': are their assumptions confirmed by what happens with other people? Almost always they're not, so they can readjust their thoughts. We encourage them to try out new patterns of thought.

We get the person to reschedule their day, structuring time for distraction from their negative thoughts and encouraging pleasurable and nice activities. Then there is activity scheduling, getting people to do things that give them some pleasure rather than the same old things.

This can be difficult to do when someone's depressed: they can see no point in it, they think they're bad and don't deserve it. We make up a list of graded tasks starting off with something fairly simple like spending more time having your hair done, or looking around your favourite bookshop.

It's important to make these tasks achievable and small. Gradually we build up to bigger tasks, and then we get people to re-evaluate some of their assumptions. This is a very powerful way of questioning the sort of negative, depressive thoughts and beliefs that they've got so stuck with.

Sometimes, it's important to include some social skills training. This consists of some basic simple ways of communicating with other people, of making friends. If people are very shy, it can be difficult for them to try out some of those big new ideas that they've now got.

Neurolinguistic programming

Neurolinguistic programming (NLP) is an intriguing form of self-development, started in California in the 1970s. It is described as 'a way of making your experiences more pleasurable, your communication more effective and rewarding, your influence more widespread, and your beliefs more contextually appropriate.'

The process sounds rather like cognitive behaviour therapy, as it consists of learning (or 'programming yourself') to change your own, unsuccessful, preconceived notions and assumptions, and to replace them with more positive and successful ones that then help you solve your problems. It is commercially promoted as a tool for business, management, education, training, and therapy (and even seduction).

Some of its proponents clearly consider it is something that will magically transform every aspect of our lives. There is a current vogue for it, and costly courses are advertised in the press. However, there is no evidence that it is effective in treating depression, unlike cognitive behaviour therapy. Also, there is no money-back guarantee with it.

Interpersonal therapy (IPT)

This is a psychotherapy developed in the USA specifically to help depression. Since it was started, its uses have spread to helping people with many problems as diverse as bereavement and eating disorders. It is a brief therapy – usually involving less than 15 sessions. It has been shown to be cost effective and helpful, and has held up well to the scrutiny of research.

The therapy focuses very much on the 'here and now', with less emphasis on the past. Current stresses are examined. The key people involved in the stresses are looked at. What are the current disputes or disappointments? Are there signs that you are learning how to cope with the situation, or that you are very stuck? What assets do you have? Depressed people are *very* bad at recognising their assets. The therapist will help you talk about difficult and painful emotions. This can lead to an examination of how you can clarify, and make known your wishes to people around you. This should lead to a more satisfying and rewarding relationship, and less negative and depressive messages being given out. 'Misinformation' can be clarified, and the therapist will try to suggest alternatives. Overall, what the therapy does is to look in depth at the way you yourself interact with other people – especially in your current key relationships, and to how this can be used to good, and sustaining, effect.

6
Alternative (complementary) medicine

In this chapter we explain what these terms mean, and discuss the results of the recent House of Lords' enquiry into the value and quality of these treatments in general. There is good evidence about one particular herbal remedy for the treatment of depression – St John's wort – and we discuss its benefits, its potential interactions and adverse effects.

We look at light therapy for seasonal affective disorder (SAD), and discuss whether there is any evidence that special diets or food supplements can help. Reflexology, aromatherapy and hypnotherapy are mentioned, and we explain what acupuncture can do – and why it won't work so well if you are suffering from depression.

What's the difference between alternative and complementary therapies?

Nothing! The term complementary is perhaps preferable (often charmingly mis-spelt as complimentary, which makes it sound flattering!), since it's very important that depression is treated in the conventional way. You may choose to add on (complement) these approaches to your conventional treatment. It is better not to use them as alternatives to medical treatment, whether this is medication or counselling/psychotherapy. Untreated depression can go so badly wrong.

There is strong scientific evidence that conventional treatments work, but there isn't any such evidence about most
complementary/alternative therapies. That's not to say they don't
have some effect, just that they wouldn't be a sensible first
choice. If taking a complementary treatment at the same time as
your standard treatment improves your general well-being, of
course that will help too (but remember that St John's wort
shouldn't be taken at the same time as other antidepressants).

About a fifth of adults in the UK used some sort of
complementary treatment in 2000, according to a recent House of
Lords inquiry on the subject. The inquiry described three main
groups of treatments:

- the 'principal disciplines' including osteopathy,
  chiropractic, acupuncture, homoeopathy and herbal
  medicine;
- the 'complementary' treatments of aromatherapy,
  hypnotherapy, reflexology, flower remedies, and shiatsu;
- the alternative disciplines of crystal therapy,
  anthroposophy, iridology, traditional Chinese medicine and
  Chinese herbal medicine.

We will discuss whether some of these methods help
depression further in this chapter, but it's fair to say that there are
only anecdotal claims as evidence for many complementary
treatments in depression. They are often expensive.

While the House of Lords report didn't condemn these
treatments, it did point out that there is a serious need for better
quality control of all complementary treatments. Their opinion
was that evidence about safety and efficacy, labelling, and
training and regulation of practitioners was all poor. If people are
to use these treatments (and some of them are pretty big
business), they should be available to the same quality and safety
standards as other more conventional treatments. Much more
research is needed (and it is difficult to find funds for research
into alternative medicine).

Herbal remedies

Surely a herbal remedy is safer than a conventional drug?

This isn't true alas. Many herbal remedies have potent effects, and of course some herbs are even poisonous. It seems to be a rule of life that there are no effects without side-effects. Most of the medication available a century ago would have been herbal remedies: opium from poppies, digitalis from foxgloves, senna from sennapods, quinine from cinchona bark, for example. Conventional pharmacology and herbalism only grew apart in the 19th century when drugs like aspirin started to be manufactured in factories on an industrial scale.

At present, herbal remedies are not subject to the same quality and safety controls as conventional drugs, even though they may have harmful interactions and side-effects. They should be better regulated.

Herbal remedies are at rather a disadvantage when it comes to research. Many safety checks and clinical trials on animals and volunteers have to be carried out before a new drug can be licensed. It costs many millions of pounds to test and launch a new drug on the market place, and it would be hard for a pharmaceutical company to recoup their investment in something that can't be patented, like a herbal remedy.

Are there any herbal sleeping remedies?

Valerian is said to have a mild relaxing effect. If you would like to try medication that doesn't need a prescription, you can buy Phenergan, a mildly sedating antihistamine over the counter from a chemist.

St John's wort

Are there any herbal remedies for depression?

There is now good scientific evidence that extracts of a herb called St John's wort are as effective as imipramine, a standard conventional antidepressant drug regarded as a benchmark for comparison in antidepressant medication. Some of the research is a little dubious, but there is evidence that it can be effective in mild to moderate depression, if taken in adequate dosage.

Why can't my doctor prescribe it then?

At present it hasn't been included in the British National Formulary as a licensed medication. More work is needed on which ingredient of the plant is the active one; there are several active compounds.

What exactly is St John's wort?

Its Latin name is *Hypericum perforatum*. A shrubby plant producing yellow flowers, it's also known as goatweed and klamath weed. It is said to flower on the birthday of John the Baptist, 24th June. First described as a herbal remedy nearly 2 millennia ago, it's been used as a folk remedy since the Middle Ages against infectious diseases (TB, syphilis, worms, dysentery and whooping cough) and also nervous complaints.

Mainstream medical interest in it was reawakened in the 1980s with published research describing benefits for people with depression, anxiety and insomnia. Its active ingredients seem to be hypericin and pseudohypericin, which are weak MAOIs (monoamine oxidase inhibitors), and hyperforin, which inhibits the uptake of serotonin, dopamine and noradrenaline, as well as GABA and L-glutamate (the brain's neurotransmitter molecules). This gives it a broader base of antidepressant activity than any other antidepressant drug. Most other antidepressants act on one of these neurochemicals.

Interestingly it is also being researched as an antiviral drug for AIDS patients. Its use for menstrual cramps has been described for over 2000 years.

I'm on the Pill. Can I take St John's wort?

St John's wort can make the oral contraceptive pill *ineffective*. You will need to discuss this urgently with your GP or family planning doctor.

Someone said I should wear dark glasses while I'm taking St John's wort. Is this true?

Not exactly, but St John's wort does cause you to become very sensitive to the sun, and you will certainly get sunburn much easier when on it. There are one or two reports in the research literature of cataracts forming in people using this herbal remedy, perhaps, just perhaps, owing to the same effect on the lenses of the eyes. This finding is certainly only at a research level and may not turn out to be more than a chance finding. More research is needed.

So does St John's wort have any side-effects?

In the clinical trials, fewer people experienced side-effects than on the conventional drugs, and fewer had to drop out of the trials owing to these. The main down-side is that it does cause photo-sensitisation: your skin becomes extrasensitive to the sun, and users should be particularly careful in the summer months to cover up and use sunblock.

It can also interact with other drugs. It induces liver enzymes, in particular the cytochrome P450 enzyme system, which means that levels of certain other medications will be reduced if you are taking St John's wort. The commonest is probably the oral contraceptive, but warfarin, and drugs used for asthma and HIV treatment are also involved.

Some of the really complex medications used for transplant patients also interact, and there have been reports of transplant rejection in people who have not mentioned that they were taking

St John's wort after a transplant. It's a herbal remedy so there is unfortunately no regulation that these interactions should be on the label. Conventional prescriptions nowadays have to include a slip with information about any possible side-effects and interactions. See the list below for drugs that might interact with St John's wort.

Like some antidepressant medication, St John's wort can provoke mania (severe excitement) in people with a tendency to bipolar illness (manic depression). Reduced sperm motility and effects on egg cells have also been mentioned in animal experiments.

Shouldn't everybody try this themselves before using conventional antidepressants?

Almost certainly not. People who have become even moderately, let alone severely, depressed should really be in touch with their doctors for their own sake, rather than just treating themselves. Depression often reduces our own insight and we may not realise how unwell we are, when an outsider would notice something wrong at once.

Herbal extracts are not manufactured to the same standards of consistency in some cases as conventional remedies, nor are they regulated in the same way. How can you be sure you are getting the right dose?

Some researchers say that the late flowers contain more active ingredients and are more effective than herbs gathered earlier in the season, so different herbal products may vary in effectiveness. This could explain why some trials didn't demonstrate benefit, yet others did.

There are potential drug interactions with some prescribed medication. Your pharmacist should be able to check this out for you, though a herbal supplier may not be aware of this. See our list below.

Avoid St John's wort if you are taking any of these:

* warfarin (an anticoagulant, used for heart and circulatory problems)

- the oral contraceptive pill
- cyclosporin (used to prevent rejection after liver or heart transplants)
- certain drugs used for HIV (AIDS treatment)
- some anticonvulsants used for epilepsy: phenytoin, phenobarbitone, carbamazepine (also used for neuralgia and mood disorders)
- digoxin (used for heart failure)
- theophyllines (used for asthma)
- triptans (used for migraine), e.g. sumatriptan (Imigran), naratriptan (Naramig)
- any SSRI.

Light therapy for SAD

Seasonal affective disorder is discussed in Chapter 2.

I do get quite depressed during the dark winter months. Medication helps but I don't want to take it every year. What else can I do?

The newer antidepressant drugs (SSRIs) have been found to be effective for SAD, whereas the older tricyclic antidepressants (TCAs) *might* make people even sleepier. Our environments change during the winter in various ways that may affect us; for example, we may have less opportunities for enjoyable sport or hobbies, our jobs may become more difficult, and Christmas can be stressful.

There is now fair evidence that light treatment is as effective as antidepressant medication for *some* people. The Swiss health service now provides it as a treatment. The American Sleep Disorders Association also recommends its application for disturbed sleep rhythms among shift workers, or from jet lag, Alzheimer's and ageing. Seasonal factors may affect people with various types of depression, and some experts suggest everybody with depression should at least try light treatment as well as their usual treatment.

What exactly is light therapy?

Light stimulates our nervous systems, and alters our circadian rhythms (body clocks). The average office has a light intensity of about 500 lux. In contrast, a bright summer's day has about 100,000 lux. Lightboxes are available commercially that produce about 10,000 lux and cost from £100 to £300. The published research has been done with this sort of equipment. You need to sit about an arm's length from it for 30–90 minutes daily, depending on the size of the lightbox. That's quite a long time! Users treat themselves through the winter months. So far, only a few psychiatric units provide this treatment.

You can also replace domestic lightbulbs and strip lights with 'full spectrum' lighting, which simulates natural daylight, but it would be difficult to light a whole room to 10,000 lux comfortably.

Are there any side-effects?

Yes. Some people get headaches, eye strain, restlessness and even insomnia. It is best used earlier in the day if this happens. You should take advice about it if you have eye disease. Too much light treatment may cause mild hypomania in people with a tendency to bipolar illness.

Who can tell me more about this?

Try the Seasonal Affective Disorder Association (SADA), whose details are in Appendix 1.

Diet

My friend is a vegan and insists my depression will be better if I go on an exclusive diet. Is she right?

No she isn't. There is no evidence that exclusive diets help depression, and some of these diets are worryingly low in certain nutrients. The best dietary advice is to look after yourself generally. Food is a basic human requirement and can give us pleasure and comfort.

- Make sure you are getting good nutrition.
- Avoid too much junk food.
- Enjoy what you are eating.
- Don't stuff yourself.
- Give yourself an occasional treat.
- Avoid faddy diets at all costs.
- If your appetite is poor, try eating little and often or 'grazing'.

What other alternative remedies can help depression? What about vitamins and health foods?

There are many herbal and vitamin supplements on sale. The health food industry is enormous, and makes all sorts of wonderful claims for its products that are mostly unsubstantiated. Unless you are seriously ill and malnourished from some physical illness, such as major bowel surgery or as a result of being on an extremely exclusive diet, there is no evidence at all that any health food supplements will treat depression. That may sound rather a crushing thing to say, but these foods and vitamins are not cheap and your money can be better spent on something that can give you or others pleasure.

Vitamins and health foods absolutely do not treat depression but, of course, there are situations where some of them can be helpful to your general health. Middle-aged women are sensible to take a calcium supplement for their bone health, such as cod liver oil capsules. People who have been heavy drinkers may need thiamine, one of the B group of vitamins. Iron deficiency anaemia can make you tired and low, and will respond to iron supplements (but note that many multivitamin preparations do not have enough iron in to be useful).

Vegan diets can be healthy but you have to be quite careful to get enough calories, iron and vitamins A and D included. Every vegan must take a B_{12} supplement to prevent spinal cord degeneration. A good source is Marmite, which is made from yeast and therefore is not an animal product.

There is some evidence that there is not enough selenium, a trace element, in UK-grown vegetables, and a supplement of this may help prevent some cancers, but there is no evidence about its relationship to depression.

There is no clear evidence that zinc supplementation helps depression.

Alternative modes of treatments

Are there any other alternative treatments that help depression? What about reflexology and aromatherapy?

Reflexology and aromatherapy are extraordinary parts of complementary medicine. We cannot explain how they could work, but depressed people can feel better in various ways after this sort of treatment. All sorts of claims are made about them but there is no firm research evidence yet.

Many sorts of physical therapy can give you a feeling of well-being. Looking after yourself, pampering yourself, reminding yourself how special you are, is always good news, especially important if you are feeling low and your self-esteem is down. A foot massage and a soothing bath with some perfumed candles will help you relax physically, and when your body relaxes your mind can too.

One special thing about complementary practitioners is that they do have time to spend with you. Having another person pay you close attention for half an hour or more can be a real change from worrying about other parts of your life and other people. A word of caution: alternative medicine is now big business. Many of these therapies are not cheap, and can be a drain on your finances.

How about acupuncture?

This is a pretty potent sort of therapy, developed in China and used for (probably) several thousand years. It consists of having very thin sharp needles put surprisingly deeply into various trigger points (called meridians) around the body. It probably works by interrupting pain pathways, and releasing endorphins (naturally occurring opiate compounds) within the area stimulated by the needles, which are left in place for a few minutes.

Besides being carried out by traditional practitioners for a variety of symptoms, it is a well recognised part of mainstream NHS treatment for a number of chronically painful medical conditions in hospital Pain Clinics.

Most Western-trained doctors wouldn't try to treat depression with acupuncture – we mainly use it for pain and stiffness problems. There is some evidence, not yet very clear cut, that it may help mood problems in conjunction with medication. There is also some evidence that ear acupuncture helps people withdrawing from an addiction, possibly by releasing those endorphins. Some drug treatment centres are starting to offer this as an alternative treatment.

Traditional practitioners of acupuncture may well try to improve general well-being with their treatment. There is no evidence that this would be an effective treatment for depression on its own, but it is safe to use with conventional treatments.

Laboratory research does suggest that acupuncture is far less effective if the subject has depleted levels of the 5-HT neurotransmitters. This suggests that it cannot work nearly so well on depressed subjects. Antidepressant treatment corrects this chemical imbalance and should enable the needles to work.

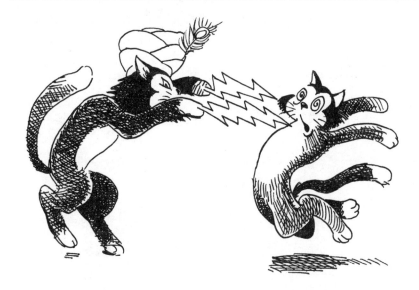

Does hypnotherapy work?

It is a very effective treatment for anxiety and tension (see Chapter 10). It can induce deep states of relaxation, although some people seem to be surprisingly resistant to its effects. Others are very suggestible and can be put into a hypnotised state very easily.

You can learn to use self-hypnosis as a way of inducing a relaxed state of mind at times of stress and tension, or just to wind down after a busy day. It does not treat depression though, nor should anyone claim it would.

7

Hospital treatment

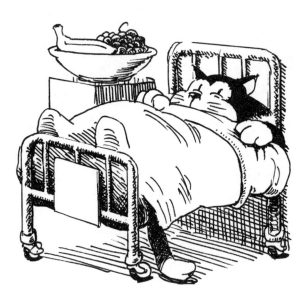

Depressive illness as we have seen, is common and very varied in its severity. Sometimes hospital admission is necessary either because the ill person is unable to care for themselves and risks serious physical harm by self-neglect, or there is a risk of harm by suicide.

The majority of people who are admitted to hospital with depressive illness are admitted with their total agreement. Occasionally, depressive illness may need to be treated in hospital without consent, and they are admitted under the auspices of the Mental Health Act compulsorily. The decision is never taken lightly, and has to be made by three professionals (two doctors and a social worker) who all agree that this step needs to be taken in the overall best interests of the person who is ill.

Quite often, after treatment has been instigated, and the person has improved enough to be able to cooperate, their status within the hospital is changed from a detained, to a voluntary patient.

The length of time people need to stay in the hospital for the treatment of depression has steadily decreased over the past years. Many people who are in hospital initially, have treatment continued as a day patient (going home each day after treatment). The step from being an inpatient to managing outside hospital can be much easier if this intermediate stage is available. Once day care has been completed there may then be outpatient appointments that continue at lengthening intervals as progress is made.

Compulsory treatment of someone with depression

What is a Section procedure?

Most people with depression are usually treated successfully as outpatients by their GPs or by their psychiatrists. A minority of people with depression will become so unwell that they may be at risk of coming to harm from self-neglect or harming themselves. They may be totally unwilling to go into hospital voluntarily. Under these circumstances the Mental Health Act exists to observe and treat someone with severe mental illness in hospital.

The Act states that when someone is a risk to their own health or safety, or to other people because of a mental illness, they may be taken to hospital. Different 'Sections' of the Act refer to different circumstances, hence the term Section.

Mental Health Act procedures are only carried out as a last resort. Even very unwell people can often realise and understand that they are ill and that they should cooperate with the treatment that they are being offered. However, sometimes people with depression or other mental illnesses lose their insight to such an extent that they cannot understand that their wishes to harm themselves are irrational and should not be acted upon.

When this happens, the Act may be used. The procedure involves two doctors and an Approved Social Worker. One of the doctors should preferably have known the patient in the past (such as their GP), and the other will have had a specialist training in psychiatry. An Approved Social Worker is there to represent the patient and family. The three individuals involved need to agree that someone is first mentally ill, and secondly in some way a risk to themselves or to other people because of their illness.

The two doctors and the social worker will usually meet at the person's home (although the procedure can also be done elsewhere, such as in a casualty department or a police station). A mental state examination is carried out and, if the doctors and social workers agree, the legal forms are completed. Usually the patient will then be escorted to hospital by an ambulance crew and the Approved Social Worker. If there is risk of harm, then the police may be asked to provide an escort.

Section 2 of the Mental Health Act applies for 28 days (for assessment) and Section 3 of the Act applies for up to 6 months (for treatment.) Other sections of the Act can be used by the police or in hospitals.

People who are detained under the Mental Health Act are entitled to appeal to a tribunal for the Section to be discharged. Details of the appeal procedure are given to all people who have been detained under a Section of the Mental Health Act. People may be allowed home on leave while still under a Section of the Mental Health Act, once they start to improve.

Can the police take you away if you're behaving strangely? One of my neighbours sometimes acts in a very disturbed way in his back garden, and I'm worried that she will upset my children.

An Englishman's home is his castle and, just because someone's very odd, peculiar or eccentric, that doesn't necessarily mean that they are ill, or that we can intervene in their lives, however helpfully concerned we are. Someone may be quite unwell mentally but, as long as there is no risk, the health and Social Services have no statutory ability to treat them. Someone who is aggressive or even violent will not come under this Act, unless they are also ill mentally.

You can discuss your concerns with your neighbour's GP if you know the practice, with the local Social Services Department (contact the Emergency Desk if there seems to be a crisis) or, in an emergency, contact the police by dialling 999.

If someone does appear to be very disturbed in a public place, the police do have powers under the Mental Health Act to take them to a Place of Safety, usually a police station, or perhaps an Accident and Emergency Department. This is known as a Section 136 procedure.

My uncle has diabetes and really bad circulation, and the doctors say he needs surgery or he may lose his foot. He refuses to consider this. We know he's going to go downhill if he doesn't have this done. Can he be made to have his operation? If he refuses, we fear the worst.

No, he cannot. Medical or surgical treatment cannot be given to people against their will, however much we feel that they need it. After all, it is his health and nobody else's.

If someone is unconscious or so ill that they cannot voice an opinion, then doctors do have to make treatment decisions for people. This may be based on Common Law (and common sense). However, if your uncle is well enough to voice an opinion about his treatment, in general we have to respect his wishes, however wrongheaded we may feel he is being. The Mental Health Act can't help us in these circumstances; it applies *only* to people who are mentally ill, and is for treatment of their mental illness, not physical illness.

In this sort of situation people are often scared of what's happening to them. Rather than a head-on confrontation, you'll get further with him by being patient and accepting how frightened he must feel. Once this is accepted and recognised, he *may* be able to start to think about what is the best thing to do.

If my husband is sectioned under the Mental Health Act, have I got to sign any papers?

No. The Approved Social Worker (ASW), together with the GP and the psychiatrist will complete the paperwork without your needing to be responsible for signing anything. ASWs are very respectful of relatives' concerns about not being put in the position of being part of a Section procedure, which could perhaps cause resentment later.

Most people who are detained compulsorily under a Section procedure usually appreciate afterwards, when they are better, that they were pretty unwell at the time, that their lives had gone well out of control, and that those involved had acted to protect their health, with their best interests at heart.

Hospital staff

What is a psychiatrist? Are they the same as psychologists?

A psychiatrist is a medically qualified doctor, with a special interest and further training in (psychiatry) dealing with emotional and behavioural disorders and mental illnesses. They are generally based in hospitals and will look after outpatients from the community as well as hospital inpatients. The most senior grade is a consultant, who will be responsible for a team of doctors, which may include Senior Registrars, Registrars, and Senior House Officers (known as SHOs), Clinical Assistants or Hospital Practitioners (who may be GPs with a special interest in psychiatry working part time in hospital), and Staff Grade doctors. University Departments of Mental Health use a different naming system, with Professors and Senior Lecturers at the top.

Psychiatrists will have a basic medical degree, plus further qualifications such as MRC Psych (Member of the Royal College of Psychiatrists). They may have a variety of other letters after their names as well – for example, if they have worked in a research post or have taken further qualifications in another branch of medicine.

Psychology is the study of behaviour, and covers memory, thought, aptitude, intelligence, learning, personality, perception and emotion. Clinical psychologists work in many hospital- and community-based teams, and will take part in a variety of 'talking treatments', such as psychotherapy and cognitive behavioural therapy. They may specialise in the assessment of people's mental ability in many situations, including dementia or following head injury. They take a degree in psychology at university, and then go on to do postgraduate training in clinical psychology, the application of the science of psychology to mental illness.

Going into hospital

I have been referred to a hospital specialist. I am not keen to see them. Do I have to go?

No, but remember that NHS resources are scarce. Your GP will not refer you to a specialist lightly. Do go to the appointment if this has been arranged. If you are not clear why your GP wants to refer you, do ask. If you are still unwilling to go to the appointment, please let the outpatient clinic staff know early. They can then offer the appointment to someone else.

Admission

Admission is suggested in less than a quarter of those being seen by a specialist. This suggestion will not be made lightly and means that there are serious concerns. Admission is very likely to be advised if there is a risk of suicide, or if the depressive illness is causing someone to eat and drink inadequately. Admission may be advised to enable treatment to be established quickly.

If the depressive illness seems to be 'resistant' to treatment – perhaps two or three antidepressants have been tried with poor results – a brief admission can enable an intensive review of treatment to take place. This review will include checking that no physical illness is present that may be contributing to the depression.

Sometimes admission is necessary in order to give a specialised treatment such as ECT (electroconvulsive therapy), which is necessary in a small minority of cases. Although ECT can safely be given to you as a day patient, there may be medical reasons, to do with the anaesthetic, for the doctors to suggest inpatient care. People who are older and frail, or have a medical illness like diabetes or heart disease, are more likely to be offered inpatient ECT than treatment as a day patient (see the ECT section later).

What happens when I am in hospital?

You will be thoroughly reviewed and details of your history – or details of the illness – will be taken. If you have been ill before, it will be important that the doctor knows what treatment you have had in the past – what has helped before is likely to help now. Details of your family history of psychiatric disorder will be taken. The events leading up to the episode will be reviewed. Details of your medical history will be taken.

Physical examination

You will have a physical examination and this will include checking over your whole body, taking your blood pressure and pulse, listening to your heart and lungs, and examining your abdomen. It will also include examining your nervous system – looking in your eyes with an ophthalmoscope, checking your muscle power and tone, checking for sensation, and tapping your reflexes.

Only rarely is a serious physical illness found at this stage – something which has been silent, or missed before. These checks do need to be done.

Tests

Following this physical examination, or perhaps because of something that alerts the doctor in your history, other investigations are sometimes indicated. These may include an ECG (electrocardiograph), chest X-ray, or EEG (electroencephalograph). If there have been marked problems with memory, this may be formally tested by a psychologist.

Some routine blood tests will be taken – physical illness can show itself via mental illness or at least contribute to it. The routine blood tests that are done are:

- *full blood count*: to check for the presence of anaemia, or signs of infection;
- *urea and electrolytes*: which give a good indication of kidney function;
- *thyroid function test*: the thyroid gland either slowing down or speeding up may cause mood disorders;
- *calcium levels*: high levels of calcium is a rare, but treatable cause of psychiatric illness;
- *liver function tests*: if these results are abnormal it could indicate liver disease – which may cause depression or lethargy. Sometimes abnormal results will be the first pointer to the fact that there has been excessive alcohol use. It can be difficult and embarrassing to be open about the amount of alcohol used. Alcohol is a powerful depressor of mood – it can cause depression. Alcohol may have been taken in a vain attempt to try and feel more relaxed and brighter in mood;
- occasionally, *folic acid in red cells* and *vitamin B_{12}*: low levels of vitamin B_{12} as in pernicious anaemia, can cause depression and lethargy before other things start to go wrong. Sometimes levels of folic acid and vitamin B_{12} may be low because of excessive drinking of alcohol.

A sample of your urine will be taken. This will be tested to see if there is glucose, protein or blood present. Each of these substances can indicate an underlying illness that could contribute to the depression (or, rarely, be causing it). Urine may also be screened for street drug use. The results are confidential – nobody will be contacting the police.

You will be weighed. A lot of depressed people lose weight because of loss of appetite. A rise in weight after admission is a sign of progress. Sometimes people overeat when depressed, and they may need help dealing with this. Weight on admission is a good baseline measure.

Treatment in hospital

When these basic investigations and tests have been done, a care plan is made. This is a treatment plan addressing your particular problems. A care plan involves an assessment by the doctor and the nursing staff. You will be allocated a 'keyworker' or professional on the ward, to set aside time to see you on a one-to-one basis. The keyworker is usually a nurse, but could sometimes be an occupational therapist, social worker or psychologist.

A programme or timetable of daily activity will be put together. This may include group therapy, occupational therapy (treatment through activity) and physiotherapy. Physiotherapists are skilled in the teaching of relaxation techniques as well as having a knowledge of a large range of therapeutic activity. You are also likely to have drug treatment that can be monitored closely on the ward.

Your care plan will discussed with you. It is a plan for your care so do ask questions. When you are well enough, day leave, then weekend leave, may be arranged to see how you cope outside the hospital. If all is well following a good leave, a target date to leave hospital is made. If it has been difficult to cope outside the hospital, it is a good opportunity to address those difficulties and try to ease them before trying leave again.

How can I keep in touch with my family whilst in hospital?

During your stay you will of course be able to see visitors. You may want to go off-site for a while with a visitor. Always ask staff first – they may otherwise waste valuable time looking for you.

Staff may suggest you do not go out initially because it can be unsettling, or you may just have been started on medication, the effects of which are yet to be seen.

On returning to the ward after a trip out, staff *might* ask to search you or your bag or to breathalyse you. This is a common hospital practice and is done to try and ensure that you and your environment are as safe as possible. Alcohol and street drugs are strictly banned from hospitals. Objects that could cause harm are also as restricted as much as possible when somebody is very low in mood.

Tell your relatives your timetable so that they are not waiting about whilst you are having a treatment session. Relatives can phone the ward to ask how you are. No confidential information will be given out without your permission. You are, of course, entitled to refuse to see visitors.

If you are visiting someone in the hospital and you are worried about anything that they tell you (perhaps for example about harming themselves), do tell a member of staff. Never assume everybody knows already. Two messages are definitely better than none.

Do I have to see medical students when I am in hospital?

No. You are entitled to refuse to see students. However, if you do agree, you are likely to be providing very valuable learning experiences for the student and you may well enjoy the contact. If you are an inpatient, a medical student may be allocated to you and become 'your student'. They can provide another source of human contact and help while you are on a ward. It is an arrangement whereby both patients and students can benefit. A student talking to somebody who is depressed will learn far more about the illness and how it affects people than she or he will ever learn from reading a text book.

Electroconvulsive therapy (ECT)

When is ECT used?

ECT is still the strongest and most powerful treatment we have for severe depression. It can and does save lives. Sadly, it has had a very bad press. When ECT was introduced in the early 1940s, it was undoubtedly overused. It began because some psychiatric patients, who also had epilepsy, seemed to do better than similarly ill patients without epilepsy. Medically induced fits were then shown to help patients with severe depressive illness. At that time there were no antidepressants or tranquillisers – just sedatives. People were desperate to find an effective treatment. Then it was given without anaesthetic, which made it look a frightening and fierce treatment. Memories of this (plus reminders through the media) perpetuate the bad old image of ECT. ECT is now given under strictly prescribed guidelines and is very different from its original practice.

ECT is given to people with severe and life-threatening depressive illness, and it includes those people who are not eating or drinking adequately, or who are judged to be a serious suicide risk. Some depressive illnesses cause abnormal thinking – delusions (or false beliefs). This type of depression responds well to ECT. ECT is sometimes recommended for people with resistant depression (an illness not improving after two full courses of antidepressant medication). It may be given when the side-effects of medication are risky. This may happen in the elderly or frail. It is sometimes used in serious postnatal depressive illness, because it is fast and effective. It is essential to try and gain improvements quickly in this situation. A sick mother cannot bond with her baby.

If ECT is recommended it does *not* mean that you are potentially incurable and that the doctors are suggesting a 'last ditch treatment'.

I am worried that I will be asked to have ECT when I am in hospital. Can ECT harm – or even kill you?

ECT is safe. It can be safely given to people with other illnesses, and does not clash or interact with medication. It is particularly effective in severe depression. There is no evidence that it can cause brain damage, and does not affect your intelligence or personality. The risk of dying during the procedure is about 2 per 100,000 procedures – this is the risk of having a general anaesthetic; ECT itself does not itself pose a danger. There is good and strong evidence that it prevents suicide.

What happens during ECT?

You will also be asked to sign a consent form (because an anaesthetic is to be given). A relative cannot consent for ECT on another person's behalf. Prior to each treatment, you can have nothing to eat or drink for 5 hours. This is standard pre-anaesthetic practice – for all anaesthetic procedures, not just brief ones like ECT.

You will have routine blood tests, and a physical examination (as for any other anaesthetic) before treatment.

The treatment involves having a carefully controlled current of electricity passed via both temples while you are fully anaesthetised (totally asleep and totally muscle relaxed). The amount of current used is low. The anaesthetic is brief – a matter of a few minutes. The current causes a brief and controlled seizure (or fit). The exact mechanism by which ECT works is not fully known (but then we are not sure how may drugs work either), but it does seem to increase the sensitivity of the brain to its own neurotransmitters. After the treatment, you sleep for perhaps 5–15 minutes. You may be a little drowsy, but you usually awake longing for a cup of tea within 30 minutes of treatment.

Are there any side-effects of ECT in the short term?

Yes. Headache is common – it usually is short-lived and responds to a simple analgesic like aspirin or paracetamol. There may be some muscle aches and pains – this is an effect of the muscle relaxant agent given with the anaesthetic. It is most prominent during the first or second treatment and will go away.

Memory is usually fuzzy for a time just before treatment and just after it (as it would be with any other anaesthetic).

Are there any long-term effects of ECT?

Almost certainly, no. This is a question that has been widely and very carefully researched both in Europe and the USA. It is still debated. If damage does occur, it is a result of the anaesthetic not of the actual seizure. People who were given very long and frequent courses of ECT in the past may show some memory impairment. ECT given as it is today has given rise to no discernible problems with memory. In fact, overall, of people who are equally severely depressed, those who have ECT do better than those who do not (if you test their memory some years later). The memory problems that have been reported are very difficult to evaluate. People who are depressed enough to warrant ECT generally have poor concentration – if you haven't taken in information it will not be there to retrieve. It may seem that you have forgotten something but in fact the information wasn't processed. Another complicating variable is that of medication. Some antidepressants are sedating and contribute to a feeling of poor memory.

How many ECT treatments are necessary?

This depends very much on the individual's response. The average course of ECT is about six to eight treatments. Treatments are usually given twice weekly. You may start to feel better after the first treatment – perhaps sleeping better that night, or there may be no discernible change until after the second or third treatment. Some people need only two or three treatments, others need up to 12. Treatment will be stopped when the rate of improvement levels out.

Leaving hospital

What happens when I leave hospital?

Following discharge from inpatient care, a letter is sent to your GP detailing what treatment and medication you have had, and the follow-up arrangements made, e.g. date of the next outpatient appointment. Arrange to see your GP in the week following your discharge, for a review. You will also need to get a new prescription for your tablets. You are usually given a week's supply of medicine from the hospital. It is worth taking the medication with you to the surgery to show your doctor – sometimes a hospital letter is delayed. An awful lot of tablets are white – the exact names and dosages will be needed.

Day care may be suggested – this may be anything from a morning a week at the hospital to 5 days per week depending on need. Day hospitals offer a wide range of treatment from group and individual work, to creativity sessions and anxiety management courses. A wide range of health professionals are involved in providing treatment in a day hospital.

When you are well enough, treatment will be completed in the outpatient department – a visit to the clinic at lengthening intervals, until your care is then transferred back to your GP. Fares to and from the day hospital or outpatient clinic *might* be refundable – do ask.

A CPN (Community Psychiatric Nurse) may visit you at home.

What does a CPN do?

CPNs review your progress, monitor treatment and sometimes do specific tasks, perhaps helping you gain confidence leaving the house. They may visit you if you have recently come out of hospital, or give regular medication to someone who has longer term difficulties, such as a psychotic illness.

CPNs may have a wide range of skills, and often have a variety of roles. Some will be 'nurse therapists', expert in providing treatments, such as cognitive behaviour therapy, relaxation training, or basic counselling. They may also have responsibility as 'case managers', coordinating community care (medications, benefits, day hospital, drop-in centres), enabling people with more severe illness to manage at home.

What is a care plan? My granny is in hospital and I've been invited to attend a case conference about her.

Every patient who is admitted to hospital will have a multi-disciplinary care plan made to meet overall medical and social needs. A key worker is appointed to coordinate care, and to see the plan through. For example, someone might need housing improvements, home help, meals on wheels and a supply of regular medication.

GPs, social workers, family, psychiatrists and nursing staff may all be involved in planning someone's care before they leave hospital, to see that every aspect of their case has been considered. Family may be asked to attend, as relatives' opinions and concerns are very important.

8

Having time off and getting back to work

If you are unwell with depression, it is important to know when to switch off from work for a while, as your work performance may be significantly affected even if you don't quite realise it.

We describe the basic paperwork – medical certificates, or sicknotes – that you will need if you become unable to work for a short or longer time. We explain how to get help with benefits, and the allowances that are available for people with longer term illness and their carers: Statutory Sick Pay, Incapacity Benefit, Disability Living Allowance, Community Care Grants, Crisis Loans and Invalid Care Allowances. We also mention where you can get skilled help to find your way through the complexities of the Benefits system.

After a spell of depression, it is often wise to get back into work gradually: the Therapeutic Earnings Scheme, as well as an Occupational Health Department can both be of help here. It is not always easy to know what to say to people at work, and we discuss who to tell.

Sickleave and sicknotes

How do sicknotes work?

For a short break of up to 1 week, you're entitled to self-certify. Your workplace will have a supply of self-certification forms (SC2). If you need longer than a week, your GP will give you something called a Med 3. This states your illness (perhaps in vague terms as we've mentioned elsewhere) and how long you're likely to be off sick. This can be a Final Note if you're going back within 2 weeks, or an Open Note if it may be longer. This can be as long as 6 or even 12 months for long-term illnesses.

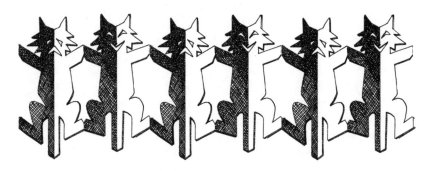

My employer asked me for a private sicknote when I was off sick for a few days. My GP says I have to pay for this. Can they do this?

Yes they can. You are entitled to submit an SC2 (self-certificate) for short spells of illness (less than 1 week) but your employer may wish for more details from your GP. This seems to happen more often when people have had a lot of sickleave. Some of us suspect that this is used as a disincentive to taking more time off work, or to make life uncomfortable for employees by discouraging sickleave. Private sicknotes cost around £10.

I missed some time off work last summer and now my employers want a backdated sicknote. Can I get one?

A sicknote cannot be backdated as it is a legal document, and today's date is today's date. To get round this, your GP can issue something called a Med 5, to state that you were indeed ill in the past. This can be done if, say, there is a recent hospital report about your case, or from GP records of your past attendances. This can be useful if you have moved, been in hospital or changed doctors. Gaps between certificates can be covered in this way, if you overlooked getting consecutive sicknotes, or if (and this is not unknown) the Department of Social Security (DSS) have lost one of your certificates.

What is a Med 4?

This completes the set of sicknotes we've described. People who have been off sick for some time must be considered for an All-Work Test, to see whether they are fit for any work, not just their usual job. The DSS may ask you for a Med 4. This gives them some more information about your state of health, and may enable them to confirm that you are entitled to longer term benefits without having to have an independent medical examination by a DSS doctor. This is usually a routine request after you have been off sick for some time.

I missed a Court attendance last week and I understand I'm in trouble. Can I be excused on medical grounds?

Try never to miss Court cases, whether as a witness or a defendant. The Bench tend to take rather a dim view of excuses. Some people with a depressive illness may become genuinely overwhelmed by being involved in Court proceedings. However, you must take action *before* the proposed Court appearance.

Talk to your solicitor about this, and ask them to write to your GP requesting a medical report. They will need your written consent for this and there is likely to be a fee. If your doctor has been treating you, he or she may be able to help, if aware of your condition, and if you would genuinely have been unable to attend Court because of it. Retrospective sicknotes are often rather difficult to do, from the GP's point of view, with the best will in the world. Make sure your GP and solicitor know with good warning, that you have difficulty in attending court.

Does your GP have to write depression on a sicknote? I don't want people at work to know about my problems.

Sadly, depressive illness is still seen by many as stigmatising. The situation is slowly improving and more and more firms – and certainly the bigger ones – will be concerned about every aspect of their employees' health, as they do have responsibilities towards your working conditions nowadays. Occupational Health Departments of the bigger firms will have a brief to improve stressful situations in the workplace, if this is a problem. If they are aware that an employee is under pressure, they may be able to alter things in the workplace to make life easier.

So, whilst in general it is best to tell the truth, there are certain cases when it is best to use less stigmatising terms. GPs will be only too aware of this issue, and are often quite prepared to write something vague and non-specific like 'Stress reaction' or 'Nervous debility' on sicknotes when necessary.

Benefits for sickness

Where can I find out what benefits I'm entitled to?

Start out by phoning the Benefits Helpline, 0800 88 22 00. Your local Social Security office will have leaflets with fuller details of all benefits. Look in the phone book under Benefits Agency for the address of your nearest one.

I'm going to have to leave my job because I have depression. What sickness benefits can I get?

My first advice is 'Don't'! That is to say, try not to make major life decisions while you are depressed. Quitting the job, selling the house, leaving the relationship are all big, long-term decisions, not to be made in a hurry. When you're depressed you tend not to do yourself justice – as your self-esteem is low (and that's part of the illness). You may sell yourself short, put other people's interests ahead of your own, and take the option that seems to cause the least bother at the time. Leaving work when you are depressed may seem OK at the time, but you may regret it when you're better.

See your GP about sickleave if you're not coping at work. Some people prefer to stay at work as they find a work routine can be soothing and help occupy the time. Some work environments are better than others, and being around sympathetic workmates, who may have been through it themselves, can be a big support. Some people seem to opt to stay at work when things are tough for these reasons.

However, some sorts of job are not conducive to this. If your job is stressful and demanding you may find that you don't make good decisions when depressed. That is the time to have sickleave for a brief while.

What is Statutory Sick Pay (SSP)?

You may be entitled to SSP from your employers for up to 28 weeks. This is paid by your employers in the same way as wages. Let them have a medical certificate as soon as possible if you are off sick.

I want to apply for a Disability Living Allowance (DLA) for my son who has been off work for some months with severe depression. How do I do this?

Disability Living Allowance is a state benefit for those people who are significantly disabled on a longer term basis (for at least another 6 months ahead) with an illness, needing major help with personal care, getting around, or both. This could include severe depression. People have to have major needs for attention (meaning help and assistance) and supervision (that means needing to have an eye kept on them) by day or by night, to qualify for this benefit.

People with some of the more severe sorts of depression could be eligible for this, depending on whether they are able to lead an independent life, or whether they need help with activities of daily living, or to see that they are safe.

Depression severe enough to need hospital treatment, perhaps with psychotic features, risk of self-harm, or needing admission under the Mental Health Act is more likely to come into this category. It is awarded on the basis of a statement made about needs. This is assessed by a civil servant, who may ask a doctor to carry out a more detailed examination. You can get the application forms from your local DSS office. There is also a Mobility Allowance component, payable if someone has problems with mobility. After the age of 65 you cannot claim for DLA but might be able to get Attendance Allowance, if you have been ill for more than 6 months.

The forms to apply for this are lengthy. An application will take at least a month to get through the system. It may be sensible to ask for help from a social worker, a Welfare Rights Worker, or the Citizen's Advice Bureau, when you are filling out an application. If your application is turned down, it may well be worth appealing or re-applying later.

My daughter had to spend some time in hospital, and hasn't been able to return to her job full time. She wants to work part-time for now. Can she get any help?

She may be able to take part in the Therapeutic Earnings scheme. This allows you to continue to claim sickness benefit, but also to receive limited earnings from working part-time. This is aimed at helping people to get back into the world of work. She needs to apply for permission to do this from the Benefits Agency who will need to ask her doctor for information.

If she is able to work at least 16 hours per week, but her earning capacity is limited by illness, she may be able to claim Disability Working Allowance to top up her income (this is a means tested benefit and will depend on her savings).

My mum is nearly 80. She needs constant looking after and we don't want to put her into a home. I've had to give up my part-time job as she needs so much attention.

If you are aged between 16 and 65, and caring for a severely disabled person who gets the middle or higher rates of DLA or Attendance Allowance, you could be eligible for Invalid Care Allowance. You would have to spend at least 35 hours a week caring for her, and there is a limit of £50 (after expenses) on your earnings. You could not apply for this if you were in full-time education.

My son has been ill for nearly a year now, and has needed hospital treatment. He is self-employed, so does not get any Statutory Sick Pay. What else is there for him?

If he's paid enough National Insurance contributions, he could get Incapacity Benefit. If he hasn't, and has been off sick for 6 months, he may be able to claim the (smaller) Severe Disablement Allowance instead.

When my daughter came out of hospital her flat had been invaded by squatters. They left an awful mess, wrecked the place, and stole all her household goods. We're doing our best to help but we can't afford to buy everything she needs.

She should apply for a Crisis Loan. This has to be repaid in the future, but anyone is eligible in an emergency, regardless of their benefit status.

If she is receiving Income Support or Jobseeker's Allowance, she could apply for a Community Care Grant, which is non-repayable, aimed at helping someone resettle into the community. Repayable interest-free Budgeting Loans are also available.

Local or national charities may also be able to help with one-off payments, to help individuals or families resettle at home. An experienced social worker or health visitor may well know of good sources of charitable help, especially where children are involved.

Isn't this a bit complicated? Who can help me sort out my benefits?

Yes, it is complicated, and you can get help. Good people to help you with benefit questions would be your Human Resources department at work, or the Citizen's Advice Bureau, a Welfare Rights Worker, perhaps your local Law Centre, or a social worker.

Can I get compensation for PTSD?

Post-traumatic stress disorder is an increasingly recognised problem after suffering – or even witnessing – some violent incident. This could range from experiencing a street mugging to witnessing the aftermath of a train crash.

If a crime is involved (a robbery or an assault, for example), the Criminal Injury Compensation Authority (CICA) make ad hoc payments to those injured in the incident. They accept that such injuries may be psychological as well as physical, and so will make payments to those seriously affected in this way. The forms are long but fairly self-explanatory. The Victim Support Scheme volunteers can help you do the paperwork to start a claim. It is always worthwhile asking for skilled help when filling them out. Solicitors will also know how this works, but remember that legal fees are not payable under this scheme, so any award would be reduced by your lawyer's bill.

Under some other circumstances sufferers may claim compensation for PTSD from third parties or employers. Careful legal advice is sensible in these circumstances.

Getting back to work

I've been off sick for a long time, and I've rather lost my confidence about returning to work. Is there any way I can gradually start part time without losing my benefit?

Inquire about the Therapeutic Earnings scheme (see earlier question) at your local DSS office. This scheme enables you to do some part-time work and receive a limited amount of earnings without losing your other benefits. You have to apply formally for this scheme and your doctor has to agree that it will help you become rehabilitated. It can be a helpful way of getting back into the world of work.

I've been off sick for nearly 6 months with depression. I want to get back to work soon, but I'm worried it will be difficult after so long.

If you have an Occupational Health Department, get in touch with them. They can help you make a planned, staged return to work if necessary. Otherwise discuss your return with your colleagues or seniors. It may be sensible to start back part time, or to shelve some of your responsibilities until you are stronger. Be aware that it may take a little time before you are able to carry your usual responsibilities. If you have any leave left, see whether you can use it up a day at a time to break up your working weeks to start off with. Having an ally at work is always good news. Try to spend more time with your particular friends for general support. Always try and go back initially midweek (the weekend will be closer!). Try to arrange to visit work before you return fully, then the 'catching up' with colleagues will have been done.

Should I tell people at work that I have been depressed?

This is a difficult issue. Unfortunately, there is still quite widespread misunderstanding and stigmatisation about mental illness. On the other hand, if an employer does not know what has been wrong with you, they may well not be able to make adjustments and changes that could be extremely helpful in your return to work. This is especially important if it is felt that stress at work has contributed to your illness. You may be pleasantly surprised by the reaction, if you do decide to confide in a trusted workmate.

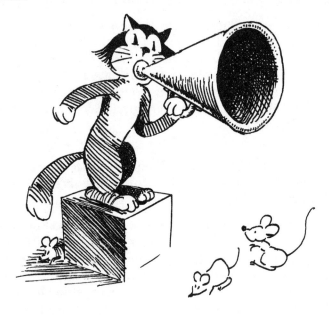

Employers now have a duty of care towards their employees – they are not permitted to subject people to the same stresses that led up to their illness. If they do expose people in this way, they are liable to be prosecuted. It is very important that your Occupational Health Department at work know the full picture about your illness, since they cannot work in your best interest if they do not know what has been wrong. The general rule is never lie to an employer about illness, but this is not the same as always telling everything. Mental illnesses are generally covered by the Disability Discrimination Act. Some, e.g. addiction, are not.

I want to get a mortgage. Should I mention having had depression on the medical form?

Strictly speaking, yes. The mortgage company may ask your GP for a medical report from your past record and, if a significant condition that you have not disclosed comes to light, they may increase your premium or decline your business. However, many people have been treated for depression and other stress-related conditions at some time in their lives – it's a common condition.

Life insurance companies are primarily looking for major risks to your health (and hence your fitness to pay back their loan), such as high blood pressure or heart disease, rather than day-to-day ills. Of course, you do have the right to see any medical reports before they are sent to the insurance company, and to alter details you don't agree with. Rather than putting 'depressive illness' on an insurance form, an answer like ' 2 weeks off sick with stress reaction' (or 'effects of stress') may be less alarming to others.

What are Occupational Health doctors? How can they help me?

Many large firms and organisations supply occupational health services to their staff. Perhaps a quarter of the country's workforce is covered in this way. Occupational Health doctors are independent of employer and GP, and have special experience in work-related illnesses. Some of the ways in which they can help include helping someone start back at work in stages after a spell of sickleave, suggesting a change of work pattern or department, and advising part-time working or using flexi-time.

They are experienced in advising managers on how to help the job fit the individual, and in finding ways to reduce not only the physical demands of a job but also the mental stress and strain. If workplace stresses contributed to your illness, your employers are not permitted to subject you to the same stress. Occupational Health doctors can also give advice about the Disability Discrimination Act. Employees can usually refer themselves directly if an Occupational Health service is available.

9
Self-harm – difficult times for you and your family

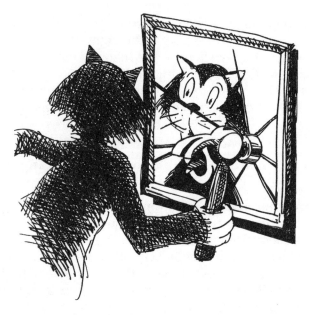

Depressive illness is debilitating and exhausting for the sufferer. It also has a very powerful effect on carers and loved ones. It is difficult to go on caring and being positive in the face of continuing negativity and inertia from the person who is ill – no matter how much you love them.

It is terribly important to recognise that carers and loved ones need care too. It is vitally important that the carer cares for themselves – it is not selfish, it is essential. You cannot help if you too become ill. You need strategies to cope.

If you are the person who is ill, you very much need strategies. Treatments – talking or drugs – do not work instantly. It may take 2–3 weeks before treatment starts to make an impact. You need to be able to cope day to day. Different strategies will work better at different times. Some of the suggestions that follow will help you, others may not and may even irritate you. Find what works for you and keep using it. Regular exercise may be enjoyable and helpful for some, for others it would a miserable trial. You need your own special recipe.

Motivating yourself is very difficult when you are depressed. Feeling pleasure often has to be relearned – it cannot happen to order. Experiment and try to be patient with yourself. When very depressed, coping with the day ahead is a very big challenge – tackle it in stages. Perhaps you need to plan ahead just until coffee time or lunchtime. The day ahead may seem very long if you see it as one big stretch of time. Try and have a mixture of things that may really have to be done interspersed with something that could possibly give you some pleasure. Pace yourself and praise yourself. Recognise that coping with the day, is a big achievement in itself when you are very low.

Dealing with someone with depression

My sister's become a real recluse. She's dropped out of her career, seems awfully depressed, doesn't look after herself, and has become isolated from her friends. We help out with money when we can, but she gets resentful if we 'interfere'. Should we leave her alone?

It sounds as though she needs help. We have all got the right to do what we want with our lives, and there is nothing to stop her leaving her chosen job or career, but this sounds more serious. If someone drops out of their chosen path and takes up some alternative lifestyle, the decision has to be accepted.

However, if they are unhappy and seem ill, it is different. Is this an alcohol- or drug-related problem? If you think so, you may start with some support and advice from your local advisory centre. These problems will affect the whole family.

This does sound more like a depressive illness and may be quite severe, so first of all, keep in touch. Don't give up on your sister, but make sure that you keep up a friendly contact. Putting too much pressure on her may be counterproductive, and people may understandably become resentful of direct advice.

Occasional lunches out, and visits to the shops together; or perhaps doing things that you used to enjoy doing together when you were younger, may be a good start. Too much pressure, on the other hand may make her resentful and she may retreat into her shell.

When she realises that you accept that she is feeling low, try to look at it together with her. Understand that people with depression feel that things can never ever improve, whatever anyone says or does. Quite often, no matter how fixed the ideas someone has, there is usually a small part of them that will accept that something is wrong, and they will want to do something to get better.

Maybe try leaving some leaflets about depression and mental health around (or a copy of this book). You may be able to get her to accept a visit to the GP with you, to explain your concerns. She might use one of the phonelines for people with mental health problems. If she won't consider medication from the doctor, she could try St John's wort as a starter, which is an effective herbal antidepressant. At least she will then be starting to address the problem.

A family member gets very depressed. We all love her but we don't know how to help, she seems so low sometimes. How can we help her?

It's really important that you help her to get started with treatment. Start out by saying that you're worried, and get her to attend the doctor's. Suggest she has a 'checkup'. Perhaps have a word with her GP. Go along with her for her first visit, if you can. It's a big help when families do this because then we know who's giving support, and we often get a better picture of how extensive the difficulties are. The doctor can never disclose the contents of a consultation with a third party, however worried and helpfully concerned you are but, if you are in the room during the consultation, you can have a three-way discussion and you will then be reassured that everything has been addressed.

When she starts on treatment, it will be helpful if you can encourage her to stay with the treatment until it really starts to work. Keep an eye on her medications to reassure yourself that she is taking them. Progress may take several weeks.

If she is not getting better, or you are worried, encourage her to say so to her doctor. Different treatments may be needed if no improvement occurs. A change in her medication or a further opinion may be helpful. About 1 person in 8 or 10 may drop out from their initial antidepressant treatment owing to side-effects, and a similar proportion will need referral to a psychiatrist about their depression.

The commonest side-effect of the SSRIs is probably initial nausea and indigestion feelings. These pass off with time, so tell her to be patient, unless they are really awful, in which case her GP needs to know. As a family member you are well placed to offer vital support. This can need lots of patience, understanding and affection. Don't give up! Talk to her and listen carefully. Realise that she may be full of low and negative thoughts, which she cannot get into perspective. These thought cycles can almost seem to be catching. Depressed people can radiate gloom in an infectious way. This can be quite exhausting to the listener. Don't be annoyed by her repeating the same worries, but do gently help her get things into perspective

If she starts to make remarks about harming herself, pay attention. Try not to panic or overreact, but do make sure her GP knows. See that you take her along for some gentle exercise, so that she doesn't get stuck in a rut. Make sure she does not miss out on social events – the company of other people is good treatment. If she doesn't want to go out, ask another time, and keep asking – tactfully but persistently – until she says yes. Do not push her too hard, do not pester her, but do not give up either.

Try to get her to take some part – just a little – in her own interests: hobbies, sports, religion or pastimes. Do not expect too much at first, as this may make her feel guilty for disappointing you. Allow her her own space, but make sure you are closely in touch. Don't get exasperated; if she doesn't seem to be responding to your support, back off a little and try again later. Recognise, and reassure her, that she *will* get better, even if she doesn't seem to believe you now. Recovery from depression takes a number of months with treatment, and can be quite gradual, so don't become frustrated. Signs of improvement include better sleep, less early waking, less sad thoughts, and a resumption of pleasure and enjoyment in normal activities. Hope is always important.

Look after yourself too; caring for a depressed person can be very draining (see below)

Carers – looking after yourself too

Carers of people with depression can have a trying time.

- Remember not to take irritability and swings in mood too personally.
- Try to encourage self-care, rather than dependency on home helps, meals on wheels, for example.
- Don't ignore any talk about self-harm but tell your doctor.
- Your relative's personal hygiene and self-care may need firm prompting.
- Discourage plans to make big life changes.
- Look after yourself: make sure that you get support and a break from time to time.

Self-harm

What can be done to help our father? He is very depressed, and seems to think he's a nuisance to us all – he isn't, we do love him dearly. He speaks of harming himself, and won't see the doctor.

Depression can indeed lead to self-harm, even suicide, although this is a rare event considering how common the illness of depression is. Those most at risk of suicide are young males – in their early twenties – and then people approaching old age, who may have other illnesses to cope with. People with drink problems are also at increased risk of self-harm.

There is a strong likelihood that this sort of depression will respond well to treatment and, in cases like this, it is most important that you urge him to see someone. There is good evidence that medication – antidepressants – will help him. Perhaps you should start by having a word with his GP about your concerns. Try and take him to see the doctor for a 'checkup'. This can be a way of making initial contact. An old person talking about harming himself is a very serious sign; however much you empathise with their loneliness and other health problems, ask for help.

My sister says she gets feelings sometimes that she wants to harm herself. What can I do?

Many people, perhaps even most people, have at some time thought about suicide, however briefly. So perhaps this feeling is at one end of our natural range of emotions, and in itself does not mean that you have a grave mental illness. However, when someone gets stuck and has this sort of thought frequently, persistently, or they feel an impulse to act on these thoughts, it warrants urgent attention. A person who has persistent suicidal thoughts should have the benefit of an expert psychiatric assessment, on the same day if necessary.

Depression can make you quite subtly lose your natural insight, and irrational thoughts and ideas can become stronger and more

Dorothy Parker, the New York poet, suffered from depression all her life. Despite two suicide attempts in her youth, she died of a heart attack aged 74. Her poems and journalism are still a joy to read nowadays, especially if you enjoy your wit acidic.

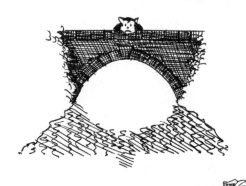

Resume

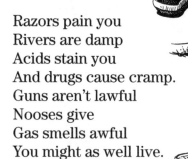

Razors pain you
Rivers are damp
Acids stain you
And drugs cause cramp.
Guns aren't lawful
Nooses give
Gas smells awful
You might as well live.

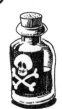

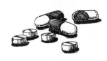

Dorothy Parker

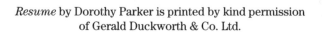

Resume by Dorothy Parker is printed by kind permission of Gerald Duckworth & Co. Ltd.

real. At the same time, people's self-esteem and self-worth become lower, so there is less to protect you from these negative thoughts. Some people with severe depression experience thoughts about self-harm becoming so strong that they appear to be in the form of voices. That is a serious matter and someone like this is at real risk of coming to harm. They need urgent assessment and treatment.

My teenage granddaughter has started cutting her forearms. She has been quite dismissive about it. Is this dangerous?

Death by wrist cutting is very unusual, but cutting as a form of non-fatal deliberate self-harm is not uncommon. Deliberate self-harm (tablets or cutting) may occur in up to 1 in 500 of 15–24-year-olds. It is more common in girls than boys.

Most people who deliberately self-harm have symptoms of psychological distress, but psychiatric illness is present in less than one-third of them.

Cutting may be a way of releasing a feeling of great tension that has built up. It could be seen as a coping mechanism – albeit an unpleasant and risky one. Cutting can become almost addictive (because of the release of tension it supplies). It might be part of other addictive behaviours such as taking alcohol or drugs. It can be part of the behaviours seen in eating disorders. There can sometimes be a background of sexual abuse. It is *not* an insignificant behaviour, and definitely warrants help.

How can we help her?

Somebody who has started to cut themselves needs help. Seeing the behaviour as a symptom of distress is very important. Sometimes families can be shocked and angry when they realise a young person has been cutting themselves. Try to resist this. Cutting is usually done in an attempt to feel better. The reason for that discomfort needs to be addressed and to be taken seriously.

My elderly aunt took five paracetamol tablets one evening. She seems upset and miserable, but my uncle says there is nothing to worry about. She has been low before and she gets over it, he insists.

You are right to be worried. The method of harm that someone uses is some guide to its seriousness, but is not a clear guide to the intent of the person taking an overdose. Most people know that taking 300 paracetamol would kill them. Not everybody knows that five paracetamol will not kill them, so your aunt's feelings around the overdose are all important. Whether or not the overdose was planned or impulsive, whether it was taken in relatively safe circumstances, or kept hidden, are also important factors when doctors assess the seriousness of the situation. Anybody who has taken an overdose, or tries to harm themselves deliberately in any way, needs to be seen and assessed by a health care professional. The action could indicate a serious suicidal intent. It is very unsafe to assume otherwise.

My sister took an overdose. The doctor who saw her in the Casualty Department said that she is not mentally ill. I think she must be to have done that.

Two-thirds of people committing deliberate self-harm are under the age of 35. It is most common in young women.

Most people who deliberately harm themselves (principally by taking an overdose of tablets) are not mentally ill. However, almost everybody who deliberately harms themselves have symptoms of psychological stress. Definite psychiatric illness is found in less than one-third of people harming themselves. However, 1–2% of those taking an overdose will die from suicide in the following year.

Deliberate self-harm is usually a measure of acute unhappiness or frustration and it is a potent way of communicating distress to the people around. Very often the overdose is taken in the setting of drinking alcohol (and sometimes taking street drugs). Alcohol and street drugs will affect judgement and increase vulnerability. Deliberate self-harm is usually impulsive.

Deliberate self-harm is usually precipitated by stressful and difficult events and is described as 'situational stress'. These events have usually occurred in the days or hours prior to the overdose (not weeks or months before). In about half, there will have been a major row with a partner or family member. There might be conflict with the police and distress of forthcoming proceedings in court. There might have been loss of a job, difficulties with money, problems with children, intolerable problems with housing. There is a big link with unemployment. There may be many, many problems, but not definable mental illness.

What can I do to help after her hospital assessment?

Take the problem seriously. Encourage her to seek help. Encourage her to see if there are any changes that can be made, or at least work towards, that will make her situation more bearable. It may be that the crisis that precipitated the deliberate self-harm is now over. It will be important to see if any everyday practical difficulties with living could be tackled and made easier – could the voluntary agencies or social services have anything to offer? A loved one taking an overdose is immensely shocking. The event can, however, be used as a starting point for important and major changes.

Suicide

Suicide is a tragic event and leaves the family with lots of unanswered questions. Box 9.1 will help in an immediate emergency.

How often does depression lead to suicide?

Suicide is sadly sometimes the outcome of depressive illness. Some people can be terminally ill with their depression. No matter what the person tries to do, to overcome their illness, no matter what help and care relatives and friends give, and no matter how skilled the medical intervention, some people will kill themselves. Suicide is totally final. It is the one solution that offers no other options, no chance for change, no future. Those left following the suicide of a loved one are left dealing with a huge range of feelings, many of which can never be fully resolved.

Box 9.1 How to get help in an emergency

Call NHS Direct (0845 4647) for general advice on how to get access to health services.

Make an appointment to see your GP, for medical help, if you need to start talking to someone who may be known to you.

Ask to speak to your GP urgently, that same day, if you feel like harming yourself.

Ask to see a psychiatrist. Your GP will usually start the assessment and treatment process. He or she can contact psychiatric help in an emergency.

Ask to speak to a CPN (or other Mental Health Team member known to you). If you are in contact with an MHT, discuss what to do in the event of a crisis. There may be a crisis line number locally, or a Crisis Team. Some people will have a crisis plan.

Call the Samaritans, if you need to talk to someone now about how you feel. (Sometimes a stranger can be easier to talk to than someone you know.)

Call 999, if someone is about to, or has already attempted self-harm, or tried to harm another person.

Attend an Accident /Emergency Department, if injuries or an overdose have occurred, or if someone appears unsafe.

Call the police, if there seems to be any risk of violence or injury occurring.

Call the Social Services Emergency Team, if you are concerned about the care or well-being of children. Approved Social Workers will also help when an urgent Mental Health Assessment is needed.

About 5000 people die by suicide in the UK each year. Most will be linked with depressive illness. The suicide rate in the UK is one of the lowest in the world at approximately 11 male deaths per 100,000 and approximately 4 female deaths per 100,000. It ranks sixth as a cause of death. There are many more deaths from heart disease, cancer, chest disease, accidents and strokes. Suicide is most common in elderly, lonely men. The suicide rate in young men is, sadly, increasing rapidly.

What sort of people kill themselves? Is there a stereotype for suicide?

Not really. It is very dangerous to assume that just because someone does not fit stereotypes they are safe. It is estimated that approximately 95% of people who kill themselves are mentally ill, over two-thirds of them will be suffering from depression and about 15% will be suffering from alcohol dependence. Men are more likely to kill themselves than women and they are normally older men – nearly half of the male suicides occur in men over 50 years old. Rates of suicide are highest in the divorced and widowed – especially the recently bereaved. Married people have the lowest death rate. Suicide is more common in the spring. Nobody is really sure why this is. Perhaps the contrast of feeling so bad, when the rest of the world is changing and growing, is particularly painful. Being unemployed and living in the city rather than the country are also risk factors.

Social class has an effect – people in the highest and lowest social classes have increased rates of suicide. It is protective to be in the middle classes. Some professions are particularly at risk, for example doctors, dentists, vets and farmers, and people working in the hotel and bar trade. Strong religious convictions lessen the rate of suicide.

Will asking about suicidal thoughts make things worse for the depressed person?

No. Asking about it can be an enormous relief to someone struggling with suicidal thoughts. It will not encourage them to act on their thoughts. If you think somebody may be thinking about suicide, always ask and always encourage them to seek help urgently.

Suicidal thoughts usually evolve fairly slowly. There can be a period of thinking in general terms about death, about how it may seem easier if, on sleeping, they never woke up. Accidents could seem to be 'lucky accidents' and a way out. These thoughts can then progress into more concrete plans. At no stage in the development of these thoughts is it too late to intervene and help. Always take statements about wanting to die by suicide seriously. Never assume that, because someone has talked about it, they will not do it.

People who talk about self-harm need to see a doctor; make sure that they do so. Talking to a friend or relative who feels like this is absolutely exhausting. Look after yourself very carefully too.

My daughter took an overdose. and was treated in Casualty. They had to wash her stomach out. It was a really horrible experience for all of us. Does such an awful experience make it less likely that she would do anything so silly again? The psychiatrist saw her and said she was distressed rather than actually ill.

Once people try to harm themselves, once they have gone that far and stepped over the limit that we all have built into ourselves, they are actually more likely to try to harm themselves again if their lives don't change. The important thing for you to do is to see that your daughter knows she has other ways of letting out her bad feelings. Talking to family and friends can be just as important as seeing a counsellor. Experiences in the Casualty Department are unlikely to stop the behaviour. The underlying difficulties and problems need to be addressed.

How do psychiatrists decide who is really at risk of suicide? How do they tell when an overdose is serious?

We have to regard all overdoses as serious and everybody who takes an overdose, however small and apparently trivial, should be assessed in hospital. People at risk include those who:

- have a diagnosable psychiatric illness, such as depression or psychosis;
- have had previous attempts at harming themselves;
- have actually caused themselves some harm;
- have other serious physical illnesses;
- misuse alcohol or drugs;
- have taken precautions against being found;
- have made preparations such as writing letters or notes;
- have made detailed plans;
- have given away possessions;
- have talked repeatedly about suicide;
- tend to be impulsive and aggressive, and
- are lonely and isolated without much social support.

The assessment after deliberate self-harm is an assessment of the balance of risk. All the above factors are examined and weighed up. This assessment is not, unfortunately, infallible.

We were terribly worried about my mother who was very depressed and tried to harm herself. She's been in hospital for two weeks and already seems much brighter now that she's started treatment. Does this mean that the risk of suicide has passed?

It is early days, and it's too soon to be sure that the worst of the risk is over. If she had severe depression, she may improve quite noticeably in the first couple of weeks of treatment, but will not be safe yet. Sometimes getting more energy and drive can actually mean that she is actually at greater risk as she might get enough drive to carry out her wish to harm herself. Talk to the ward staff who are best placed to advise you how she is progressing. It may be some time yet before they are happy to let her leave the ward, even briefly.

Will somebody who has taken an overdose go on to do it again?

Unfortunately some people will – about 15% will repeat it within the next year. There is more chance of repetition of deliberate self-harm if the episode was not obviously linked to a situational crisis or the use of alcohol or drugs. There is more chance of repetition if the person has few social supports, is in the lower social class and has been separated from a partner. There is an increased risk of repetition if there is a history of psychiatric treatment. It can be difficult sometimes to assess someone following deliberate self-harm. When people are referred to the casualty department, having taken an overdose, their medical state is dealt with and they are made physically safe. There then follows an assessment of their mental state. This is essentially weighing up the balance of risks. Another very important part of the assessment is deciding whether or not the person is currently mentally ill (rather than very distressed, without illness).

My mother had many spells of depression, and finally took a fatal overdose. What can we tell our children?

When somebody dies under tragic circumstances, such as a sudden illness, accident, or worst of all, by their own hand, then the loss is much tougher for everybody to deal with. Suicide is fortunately rare. We know that most people who do kill themselves are indeed suffering from depression (and in this book we repeatedly emphasise how important it is to have depression fully treated, because there is strong evidence that treatment can prevent self-harm and suicide). Sadly, in a small minority of cases, even when depression is treated, a depressed person will attempt self-harm, maybe fatally.

This is the sort of situation where there are no clear guidelines. You certainly won't want to break this sort of bad news explicitly to a young person unless you are sure that they need to know about it – and are able to deal with it. Mature teenagers may want to find out for themselves what actually happened, and may well resent not being told the truth.

Family secrets are difficult things to keep. Very young children may have paid little attention to the loss of their grandmother. Older children and teenagers may have heard details of what happened at the time, or they may well pick up facts later. If you do need to explain to a young person what happened, remember that this will raise all sorts of painful feelings, not least of all anger.

Family may feel deserted or hurt by their dead relative, and may feel guilty or angry about what happened – angry with the deceased person, with other family members, or with themselves. Young people may show this in different ways, by changes in mood or by difficult behaviour.

If the time does come when you have to discuss this with your family, emphasise that she had an illness, and that it was the illness that is to blame for taking her life. Remind your family to recall happy times they had together in the past, rather than today's sadness, and make sure that you are around to give support to each other.

Grieving after bereavement is a natural process that takes time. If difficult feelings are not settling as the months go by, organisations such as Cruse can help the bereaved to resolve their loss (see Appendix 1).

My father died by suicide. I badly need to talk about it but my brothers won't discuss it. What can I do?

We know that most people who die by suicide are definitely suffering depressive illness. Alcohol or drug misuse and other mental illness are also causes. Few people kill themselves without being seriously ill in one of these ways. Although your father's death was caused by an illness, just as directly as heart disease or cancer causes people to die, he has left behind survivors – family and friends – who will carry the scars of what happened to him for the rest of their days.

Depression leads people to live increasingly inward-looking lives, with less and less thought about other people. Sufferers may come to overlook the hurt that they will cause the family and act in a way that ignores other people's feelings. Your brothers are, of course, going to be shocked and distressed by his death, but this sort of death is the most difficult to grieve over. His act of suicide may seem aggressive, a direct attack on the survivors. They may well be angry at what happened: angry at him for doing it, angry at his doctors for not somehow stopping him, and even angry – and guilty – at themselves for not realising how unwell he was.

Death is our last taboo, people will talk about anything else. There is much stigma attached to someone who has committed suicide, and so it won't be easy to talk about his death outside your family. People grieve in different ways: some express themselves loudly and clearly, others deal with their grief in a quieter and more private way. Neither way is wrong. Perhaps you can make a start with them by saying that you feel angry too. If they are not ready to talk yet, do seek help for yourself from Cruse, the voluntary group skilled at helping the bereaved (see Appendix 1).

Every day I chose, sometimes gamely, sometimes against the moment's reason, to be alive. Is that not a rare joy?

Andrew Solomon

10
Anxiety states

Feeling anxious is a natural human response to protect ourselves from harm. If you're in a risky situation, your body releases adrenaline, a hormone that raises your pulse rate, opens your pupils, increases your circulation and alerts you to be physically ready for 'fight or flight'. This primitive response was very useful in the primitive world when you might suddenly have to fight off a sabre-toothed tiger or run into the jungle carrying your baby. Adrenaline gives us drive and alertness, which helps us react to any stressful situation.

Nowadays our stresses tend to be mental rather than physical ones. Home worries, relationship disappointments, family tensions, money problems, unfulfilled dreams are all sources of worry and anxiety. Sometimes these problems can be resolved and then our anxiety goes but, if left unresolved, they can cause illness. Perhaps together with an exhausting job or some physical ill-health, they can then combine to make one feel persistently anxious.

Our underlying personalities matter too. Some people have very placid unruffled personalities, whilst others are more highly tuned and sensitive. Some of us are life's worriers, others seem to take everything in their stride, but everyone has their limits and nobody is immune. We can't expect to transform our underlying personalities and change ourselves into different people, but we can accept ourselves for what we are, recognise our own potentials and strong points, and live with or work on our own weak areas.

Anxiety can be useful, or can be incapacitating and cause suffering and loss of function. The term anxiety disorder covers the mental and physical manifestations of anxiety. Anxiety can be of several types. It can be:

- persisting: a generalised free-floating anxiety
- focused: on a particular situation or animal, as in *phobia*
- overwhelming: as in *panic*.

There is a feeling of fear and this may be accompanied by a feeling of impending doom. There is physical and mental discomfort. It is a feeling about the future – what *might* happen (not what has happened). There is a feeling of threat about the situation. The emotion it causes is out of proportion to the reality of the circumstances.

My wife just worries and worries about the slightest thing. It's got right out of proportion. You can't reassure her and she makes herself ill with it.

Some of us are just 'born worriers'. One person said she had to do all the worrying in her family because, if she didn't, nobody else would. If worry and anxiety become a major part of your life, you can make yourself ill with it. The picture of an overanxious person can include symptoms such as physical tension (headaches, exhaustion, poor sleep), physical overarousal (palpitations, excess sweating), or mental tension (poor concentration, nervousness, irritability). Stresses – major or minor – may set these off, and so can too much alcohol.

Its important to avoid using tranquillisers in this situation. They may give temporary relief but, unless your wife's ability to cope changes, she will feel the need to keep taking them.

Start off by helping to build herself up, both physically and psychologically. Going to a sports club, aerobics class, yoga session or gym will relax her physically and increase her sense of well-being and self-confidence. Encourage her to do sports or pastimes that she may have enjoyed in the past.

Counsellors or therapists may use structured problem-solving techniques to help with excess anxiety. They might challenge her anxious thoughts and worries by asking her to write them down, and producing some rational solutions to them. People then choose their own best solution, and the therapist then helps them to put their plan into practice, and reviews their results.

Again, anxiety management classes, relaxation groups, or cognitive behaviour therapy are all recognised as being helpful therapy for generalised anxiety disorder. Medication can also help anxiety (see below).

Generalised anxiety

Generalised anxiety can become a problem at any time of life, but often begins in early adult life. Women are more often affected than men. Anxiety accounts for just over a quarter of the psychiatric complaints that are seen by general practitioners. About 4% of the population are affected.

You are continually apprehensive and worried. You feel tense, particularly in the muscles of the head and neck. The autonomic nervous system (outside our control) is overaroused. Part of this arousal is expressed as 'hypervigilance' – being on the alert, and scanning the environment for possible dangers. You might have difficulty sleeping, particularly difficulty in getting off to sleep, and interrupted sleep. There is a continuing feeling of 'being on edge'. It is common to feel tired with anxiety – not just because of loss of sleep, but because being on the alert for long periods is exhausting.

What causes it?

There are many factors that are thought to contribute. There is some genetic influence – anxious families producing anxious children. Past experience of separation from parents can predispose to anxiety states in adult life. There is sometimes a background of an expectation to achieve, and also conform, excessively. Then there are more obvious links, such as current

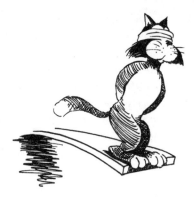

stressful situations, particularly *uncertain* situations. Uncertainty gives rise to a feeling of lack of control over one's destiny, and this is uncomfortable and draining.

Treatment of generalised anxiety

Practical intervention
When someone is troubled with anxiety, it is worth looking at very basic intervention to try and help deal with the current situations that might be causing the anxiety. Money – or its lack – may be a grinding difficulty and anxiety. Seeking help from a debt counsellor at the Citizen's Advice Bureau can transform financial chaos and worry into a manageable task to be worked out systematically.

Psychotherapy
Psychotherapy can be helpful, particularly cognitive behaviour therapy (see Chapter 5). This is especially helpful in panic disorder (see below). The question is asked, 'What are the thoughts that lead to panic?' Work is done to replace these unhelpful thoughts with more realistic thoughts. You might be asked to consider how likely it is that you really will have a heart attack if you stand up and give a presentation at work. You will be encouraged to structure your thoughts differently and replace previously anxious thoughts with more realistic and helpful thoughts.

Anxiety management training

The techniques used are clear and easily learnt. They give sufferers skills to learn, and to go on using themselves. The techniques include the use of distraction (moving on to different thoughts), the control of anxious thoughts, relaxation and breathing exercises, and education. If you have learnt about the effects of anxiety on the mind and body, the manifestations it has can be much less frightening.

Drug treatment

The old-fashioned (but still effective!) tricyclic antidepressants such as dothiepin or doxepin are efficient anti-anxiety drugs, as well as being antidepressant in action. The newer antidepressant group, the SSRIs, can be very useful in the treatment of anxiety. Both these groups of drugs are of course non-addictive, and can be taken for as long as is necessary.

Beta-blockers are drugs that are used in the treatment of high blood pressure. They can also be used in anxiety. Probably the most effective way to use them is in short bursts for helping to control anxiety (and perhaps tremor) when performing – for performance anxiety such as a musical performance or giving a lecture. They are not really so good in helping with anxiety in the long term. Another problem is that continued use of beta-blockers can sometimes cause a lowering of mood.

The diazepam family of drugs (such as Valium) is very good at reducing anxiety. However, there is a big and very important disadvantage to their use, and that is that they are habit-forming. They are difficult to stop, and their dose has to be increased over time to achieve the same result. They are useful drugs in the treatment of anxiety but they should be used for short periods only (days, or a few weeks, rather than months).

Very occasionally, when none of the above drugs is helpful and behaviour therapy has not dealt with the whole problem, the MAOI group of antidepressant drugs may be used. They are effective in severe anxiety but they do have to be used with great care. You would have to stop eating any tyramine-containing foods, the most common of which is cheese – and they have potentially very serious interactions with some other drugs. The

MAOIs are used only occasionally in the treatment of severe anxiety.

My GP has started me on antidepressants. I certainly am depressed but there are times when I experience severe spells of anxiety. She says the antidepressants will help the anxiety in time, but I wonder if tranquillisers such as Valium wouldn't help too?

Depression and anxiety are often found together. Treating the depression will lower the level of anxiety.

In recent years GPs have been increasingly cautious about prescribing tranquillisers. They were overused by the previous generation, before we became aware of their side-effects and their habit-forming potential. This can develop after only 2–3 weeks of daily use.

Some people are certainly particularly vulnerable to the habit-forming potential of tranquillisers and, if we could be clearer as to who is at risk of this sort of problem, then perhaps the pendulum of treatment could swing back a little.

Panic disorder

Recurring panic attacks can occur with no warning, although they can be linked with specific situations, e.g. an open space, a crowded shop, or heights. There is a sudden intense feeling of fear and apprehension with a variety of bodily sensations that may include palpitations, shortness of breath, sweating, faintness, nausea, chest discomfort and pins and needles in the hands and feet (sometimes around the mouth). This is such an unpleasant experience that, not surprisingly, a so-called 'anticipatory fear' develops – a fear of panic occurring and a fear of loss of control.

Approximately one-third of people who experience panic attacks are clearly clinically depressed. For the two-thirds who are not, the response to antidepressant medication is still impressive.

I had a sudden choking feeling for no reason at all at college the other day. I've had several since term started. I feel I can't breathe, my pulse races, and I think that I'm going mad. The doctor said it's not my heart, but a panic attack. What causes these panic attacks?

Some small, perhaps scarcely noticeable thought or feeling triggers anxiety. The body picks this up and reacts to it in an exaggerated way. Adrenalin is released, which raises your pulse rate and alerts you. You then perceive this and interpret it as something badly wrong, something physical. This in turn causes more anxiety and a vicious cycle results of anxiety, arousal and terror. It tends to happen to people who are highly stressed, and may occur with depressive illness, when your coping reserves are low.

People may get chest pains, dizzy attacks, trembling, sweating, palpitations, choking, or feelings of unreality and detachment. They may breathe extra fast and breathe off too much carbon dioxide from their bloodstream, causing tingling in their arms and face. This experience may be terrifying. One useful trick to stop hyperventilation is to breathe in and out of a big paper bag for five minutes. This restores the normal balance of blood gases, and will stop your hands and face tingling.

Maybe 1 person in 10 has a panic attack at some time – they are quite common. Panic attacks, although very unpleasant, do not cause lasting physical harm.

How can I deal with these panic attacks? What can I do to prevent them?

See your GP for a physical checkover, to exclude any other physical causes of these symptoms. Panic disorder can be mimicked by some medical problems, such as an overactive thyroid or disturbance of heart rhythm. Your GP may want to do a blood test and possibly an ECG.

You can help yourself by reducing alcohol, caffeine, and nicotine (all these can increase anxiety). Be particularly careful not to use alcohol as a tranquilliser. Remember it is habit-forming; it also causes rebound anxiety, i.e. later, the anxiety is *worse* than before you had the drink. Do not avoid places or situations where panic attacks have happened. This could reinforce your anxiety and make it worse. Box 10.1 gives you some advice for a panic attack.

If you have an attack:

- Do not rush off or run away (that would increase your adrenaline output and make you more excited), but stay put.
- Practise deep, controlled, steady breathing.
- Try to concentrate on some outside object rather than thinking about how you feel.
- Learning meditation techniques can help distract your mind from its own anxiety.
- Cognitive behavioural therapy (CBT) has been shown to be a good treatment.
- Consider also contacting one of the self-help organisations such as No Panic, or Triumph over Phobia (see Appendix 1).

Box 10.1 What to do during a panic attack

- Try to stay put, do not run off.
- Practise deep, slow, controlled breathing.
- Use a *paper bag* if you are hyperventilating (breathing very quickly).
- Focus your thoughts on some outside object, not on your own symptoms.
- Keep reminding yourself that it will soon pass off.

Phobias

A phobia is a focused, extreme anxiety beyond what is a reasonable response for the situation. The fear cannot be reasoned away – you cannot tell a spider phobic a spider will not hurt them, and expect them to relax. The fear response is out of your voluntary control, and it is so unpleasant that it leads to avoidance of the feared situation or animal.

Agoraphobia is the commonest phobia prompting treatment. Agoraphobia means a fear of open spaces from the Greek word *agora* for a market place. The term is also used for a fear of shopping and crowded places. It most often develops between the ages of 15 and 25 years, and may be trigged by a big life-event (such as having a baby).

Social phobia is also common. This is a persistent fear of situations where you might be scrutinised. There is often an associated fear of doing something embarrassing or out of

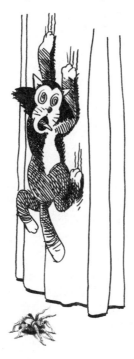

control, such as blushing, fainting or being sick. More women
than men are affected. It often begins around puberty – when
self-consciousness tends to be at its peak in all of us.

Animal phobias tend to start earlier than the other phobias.
They may start in childhood.

Treatment of phobias

Drug treatment is not usually helpful (unless there is an
accompanying depressive illness – which is not uncommon).

Behaviour therapy is the cornerstone of the treatment of
phobias – behaviour is modified with several different techniques.
If you gradually expose someone to the feared situation, and
teach them to relax at the same time, their anxiety will slowly fall
– you learn to do it without fear.

This relearning can be done gradually, or in big chunks of
exposure called flooding. The feared response is generated and
you 'stay with it'. Your body cannot sustain very high levels of
extreme anxiety for long periods – you start to get used to it, or
'habituate'.

Finally fear can be overcome by 'modelling' behaviour on the
therapist – the therapist touches a snake and shows no sign of
alarm or retreat. The patient then follows the example of
behaviour in the therapist.

All these treatments are safe and are appealing in many ways –
we know they work and they are logical with a very clear
outcome.

**I'm terrified of flying. I shake like a leaf as soon as I get
on the bus to the airport. It's ridiculous really as I'm
usually up for anything. I'm grand as soon as I get there.**

In this situation tranquillisers just for your flight there and back
can be very helpful, or some beta-blockers. Elsewhere in this
book you've seen how frightfully mean we are nowadays about
giving out tranquillisers like Valium. This sort of setting, however,
is a 'one-off'. Beta-blockers are helpful too, but they cannot be
used if you have asthma – they can make it worse. Drinking

excessively on the plane is *not* good and can compound the problem.

People who need to fly regularly for a living and have a phobia about it can be treated by behaviour therapy. Treatment involves 'deconditioning' you by gradual exposure to the source of your worry. A typical programme would involve learning relaxation techniques, and then making a series of supported visits to an airport, leading up to a trial flight.

My mum is afraid to go out of our home. She can get to the local shop, but can't get into town to see us. It's a real nuisance, and she can't go out to work. What can we do to help her?

Your mum is showing signs of a phobic condition. Agoraphobia is defined as fear of open spaces, although phobia sufferers may be afraid of people, heights, crowds, going into public places, using public transport, speaking in public, or leaving home. There are also some specific phobias.

Some sufferers may lead progressively more limited lives. These conditions can certainly be helped by treatment. Start by helping her to define exactly what she can and cannot do, however irrational it may seem. Where, or how far, can she go? Can she go to some shops but not others? Make a list so that you understand her boundaries. Start with something she really wants to do but cannot, so that she is well motivated. An example might be a visit to her favourite store to buy herself an outfit, or a Christmas present for someone.

Plan a series of small steps towards this goal: start out with a brief walk each day with someone there to reassure her. Once she gets used to this and is no longer anxious, start to do a little more each time you go out. Sometimes it can be helpful to have someone walking a little way behind when she first goes out – gradually make the distance between them longer. If she feels overwhelmed, practise some breathing and relaxation exercises with her until it passes. If she is using medication such as beta-blockers or tranquillisers to reduce anxiety, try to avoid using these while you are working on these steps (but never stop antidepressants if she is taking them). Keeping a diary record of how far you go is useful. Gradually increase this until she can reach the goal you set, first with you, then on her own.

Self-help groups can be very helpful with tackling these symptoms (see Appendix 1 for some addresses).

Since my early teens I've had what I thought were panic attacks in restaurants and canteens. My GP tells me I have social phobia. What is this condition?

Social phobia is an exaggerated and irrational fear of social situations. These can include visiting restaurants, the theatre, travelling on public transport, and 'socially dense' work situations. Although it can be considered an extreme form of social shyness, it is subtly disabling and quite difficult for others to see and understand.

Sufferers often self-medicate their anxiety with alcohol, and there is therefore a high risk of alcohol dependence. Alcohol should be discouraged, not only because of its inherent health risks, but because of rebound increased anxiety during the hangover phase when the alcohol effect wears off.

True panic attacks with hyperventilation, racing heartbeat, shaky hands, and feelings of terror or impending doom can occur in social situations. Your circulation can be affected causing fainting. You may become disabled because of panic attacks, phobic avoidance of social situations, and secondary depression.

What treatment can I have for it? The doctor suggests I try an antidepressant. Why is this?

Whether or not depression is obviously present, moclobemide (a reversible MAOI) and paroxetine (an SSRI) are licensed for treatment of social phobia. Probably all SSRIs are effective in social phobia, but only paroxetine at present is licensed for it. Besides medication, psychological therapy, namely cognitive behaviour therapy (CBT), is helpful.

How can I change my thoughts and feelings?

If your social phobia occurs in restaurants, for example, your thinking sequence might be:

- I am going to a restaurant, I am going to shake.
- I am in a restaurant, I am shaking and going red.
- I am verging on having a full-blown panic attack.
- People can see me doing this.
- They are scrutinising me, and will laugh and judge me.
- I will look a fool, be ridiculed and humbled.

CBT aims to analyse how true each of these thinking stages are, and to explore the emotions that the thoughts are associated with.

For example:

- You may indeed be shaky when in a restaurant, but how noticeable is it?
- Even if it is present, why should others be interested enough to notice?
- Even if they do notice, why should they be judgmental?

By challenging 'negative automatic thoughts' like these, initially guided by a therapist and then by yourself while in the anxiety-provoking situation, cognitive therapies aim to reduce the disability associated with social phobia.

Burnout and stress

I work as a teacher and I have had so many demands lately on my time because of a forthcoming OFSTED inspection that I just don't seem to have any go left in me and I make silly mistakes. Is this burnout?

Burnout is a popular term, rather than a clearly defined medical diagnosis. It is widely used to describe a syndrome (a collection of symptoms) of emotional exhaustion, in a context of overwork and depleted resources.

Some of the signs (in alphabetical order) are apathy, denial, depressed moods, exhaustion, forgetfulness, guilty feelings, indecisiveness, insomnia, irritability, lack of enthusiasm, loss of sex drive, loss of interest in usual pastimes and hobbies, paranoid feelings, social isolation, stress, temper outbursts, working later and later.

The term 'burnout' isn't a formal psychiatric diagnosis. It is commonly used to describe professionals, particularly those from the caring professions, who have become exhausted to the stage of indifference, perhaps in a climate of complaints and imposed changes. Once you, or a colleague, have gone this far, you may then be at risk of making all sorts of mistakes, which will cause you, and others, progressive trouble, which you then are unable to cope with. The situation can worsen.

Perhaps the best treatment is not to let it happen in the first place. Recognise the signs of stress in yourself and colleagues, and see that you step away from your pressures as early as possible. Support your colleagues if you see that they are flagging. A few kind words can make all the difference on one of those days when nothing goes right.

- Lower your horizons, accept and set some quite modest goals.
- Watch out for warning signs: irritability, not bothering, taking it out on undeserving colleagues, inability to relax.
- If you have symptoms of depression, acknowledge this and seek help.
- Take advice, and get support, from your peers and colleagues.
- Many professionals dealing with people's problems have work 'supervision'. If you don't have this available, organise it for yourself.
- One-to-one or group support can be very helpful.
- Polish up existing skills, and develop some new ones. Take pleasure from them.
- Play to your own strengths. Do what you're good at, and enjoy it.

- Reward yourself; make sure that you get away for regular coffee and lunch breaks.
- Make sure that you take your annual leave.
- Can you take a sabbatical?
- Don't neglect your family, your spare time, or your hobbies.
- Investigate early retirement, but don't give up too easily.

I'm a workaholic. All my nervous energy goes into thinking about my job, morning, noon and night. My wife and family complain, and perhaps they're right. What can I do?

Some people do really start to act as if they're addicted to their work, just as you can get addicted to harmful substances. As with other addictions, family and friends can suffer as a result. Perhaps it's a question of remembering to keep a balance between your life at work and life at home, and remembering what you really value in life. Try to invest some of your drive into activities away from work, at home or in your local community. Try and find yourself rewards outside the world of work and use some pointers from the list above.

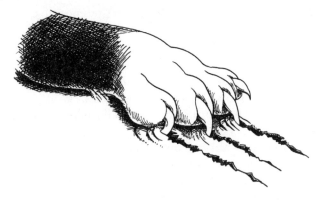

I know that, if I get too worked up about things, it really takes it out of me, and then I start to feel very low. How can I deal with stress better?

You're right to recognise that you shouldn't push yourself too far. The commonest sources of stress in people's lives are probably relationships, money, work-related issues, and family – singly or in combination. These may affect us in the form of immediate crises, or as chronic, long drawn-out worries. Boredom is also stressful – ask anybody who has been unemployed. We often have blind spots to how these things affect us. Ill health and stress do go together: we know that stress raises your blood pressure and heart rate. The symptoms of stress – poor sleep, tension, irritability, mood changes, poor concentration – if prolonged, merge into those of anxiety and depression.

Here is a list of antistress tactics:

- It's down to you; you have, in fact, more control over the situation than you think.
- Don't burn the candle at both ends; make sure that you get proper time off.
- Look after yourself properly: have a sensible diet and have proper meal breaks.
- Have an early night now and then, and an occasional late one too.
- Watch out for overuse of caffeine, alcohol, nicotine, (and other, worse, substances).
- Take some exercise regularly, just a few minutes every day is a start.
- Enjoy a creative hobby – take one up if necessary.
- Walk away from trivial disputes and disagreements.
- Watch out for signs of pressure: driving too fast, being irritable. Then slow down.
- Agree with people sometimes – you'll make some useful allies.
- Talk to someone about how you feel.
- Put something back in for someone else.
- Can you learn assertiveness skills (rather than aggressiveness)?
- Accept what you cannot change, and change what you need to.
- Plan ahead, allow yourself time for things – especially time off and leave.
- Delegate things. Learn to say no.

- Settle for 'good enough' rather than perfect sometimes.
- If you're sick, go off sick.
- Give yourself a treat sometimes.

Obsessional compulsive states

The word 'obsessional' is overused. In psychiatry it can be applied in three clear settings:

- *An obsessional compulsive neurosis* This is an illness in its own right;
- *An obsessional symptom* This can occur in many mental illnesses, e.g. anxiety states and eating disorders. People with anorexia nervosa may feel the need to know the exact calorific content of each food they are eating or cut up their food in a particular way.
- *An obsessional personality type* This is a way of describing people of particular personality who *may* then go on to develop an obsessional compulsive neurosis. To have some features of obessionalism in your character can be very useful. Obsessional people tend to be careful, do not take undue risks, check what they are doing and set themselves high standards. The negative side of this personality profile is that it means you may be less flexible, and deal less well with change – there is a need to feel in control.

Obsessions are recurring and persistent ideas, images or impulses that the person experiencing them knows are irrational and sometimes absurd. They are fully aware that the thoughts come from their own mind. They attempt to resist the thoughts and it causes suffering. The thoughts can recur hundreds of times a day.

Compulsions are the actions that a person with obsessive compulsive disorder (OCD) feel that they must, reluctantly, perform, for example washing hands for fifteen minutes after using the lavatory. There is a compulsion plus a desire to resist it (which causes mounting agitation and unpleasant tension).

There is a big overlap between OCD, depression and anxiety. Very often elements of all three illnesses are seen in OCD.

I have been told that I have OCD. What causes it?

We believe that OCD is caused by abnormalities in the dopamine system of the brain. This chemical abnormality can be seen using special PET (positron emission tomography) scans.

Can it be treated?

OCD is successfully treated with behaviour and drug therapies. As you improve, not only do you function much better but, if a PET scan is repeated, it reverses. This is an exciting finding and one of the very few illnesses in psychiatry where we can 'track' the chemical imbalance. In the future, we may well be able to do the same with other psychiatric illnesses.

Behaviour therapy is very helpful. Several approaches are taken:

- *Response prevention* is a behaviour therapy technique in which you are gently prevented from performing rituals. The therapist might also help 'model' new responses – perhaps dirtying hands and waiting a long time before washing them again. The sufferer is encouraged to do likewise.
- *Recurring thoughts* can be more difficult to treat than the actions. Thought stopping, however, can be very helpful. You need a loose-fitting elastic band on your wrist. When the unwanted thought occurs, you say 'Stop' and 'ping' the band. This stings your skin a little, and stops your thoughts. You then try breathing more smoothly and deeply; meanwhile you can either 'ground' yourself in the here and now, and look, listen and become very aware of your surroundings – the colours in the room, the feel of the chair you are sitting on, and so on. This technique pulls you back from going over and over your thought and you replace it with an awareness of your surroundings. The thought will

recur – you then need to repeat the process. If you prefer, instead of really being in the present, you can imagine (in detail) the scene on your favourite beach. You can become very skilled at this with practice. A yoga teacher can help teach this method.

- *Cognitive behaviour therapy* is much less effective in OCD than behaviour therapy.

What drugs will I be given?

Clomipramine is a long-established tricyclic antidepressant that is useful in OCD. The dose can be slowly and steadily increased as necessary. It has calming, anti-obsessional effects.

The newer SSRIs like fluoxetine (Prozac), citalopram (Cipramil) and paroxetine (Seroxat) all have anti-obsessional effects. None of the group has been found to be more effective than another, but you may find that you can tolerate one particular drug better. The dose of drug used to treat OCD tends to be higher than the dose used in depression. The anti-obsessional effect may not clear for up to 7 or 8 weeks. It is worth trying to be patient. Before the anti-obsessional effect is seen, some of the unpleasant tension, anxiety and low mood, which so often accompany OCD, may well show a good improvement.

Drug treatment and behaviour therapy are equally effective. There is, as yet, no research evidence to say that combining drug therapy with behaviour therapy is better still, but clinical experience suggests that it may be.

11
The future

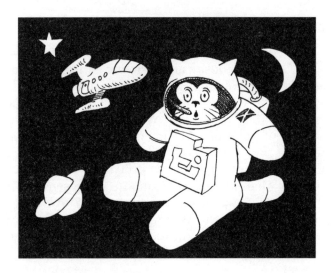

Neuroscience research is one of medicine's new frontiers. Today's latest scanners and neurochemistry labs tell us a wealth of information about how the brain actually works. Antidepressants work for most people but, like all drugs, they do have some side-effects. We can expect future generations of antidepressants to become increasingly sophisticated, more effective with fewer side-effects. We will have more choice of medication, and a better understanding of matching the patient's needs to the drug's profile.

The human genome project is helping us understand much more about the effect that genetics – your family history – has on the individual.

Research into talking treatments, counselling and psycho-therapy is more difficult in practical terms than testing out a new drug. We do have clear evidence that cognitive behaviour therapy

198

and behaviour therapy are effective treatments and they are much easier to evaluate. You can't do cognitive behaviour therapy or counselling in a test tube. The Health Service, however, recognises the importance of providing care that is both good value and effective for people, and evidence is constantly gathered and sifted to tell us which therapy is the most effective. So stronger evidence for – and against – today's treatments is always emerging.

The importance of research evidence also applies to alternative therapies. They too must be scrutinised for safety and cost-effectiveness, just as rigorously as any other medication. St John's wort is a good example of a herbal remedy that is a potent antidepressant – and which can interact harmfully when misused. It may well become prescribable before long.

Apart from newer drugs and the right sort of counselling, are there any different, more radical approaches to treatment?

Vagal nerve stimulation (VNS) and *transcranial magnetic stimulation* (TMS) are two recently invented rather remarkable methods of affecting brain function that have shown some promise in early trials for the treatment of resistant depression.

VNS involves the implantation of a pacemaker-like device in the chest wall, which is then connected to the vagal nerve in the neck. A tiny pulse of electricity is passed up this nerve into the limbic regions of the brain every 5 minutes for 30 seconds. VNS is becoming an established treatment for intractable epilepsy and is very safe. Some preliminary research has indicated that it may be an effective treatment for severe and resistant depression as well. However a great deal more research is needed.

TMS involves the application in pulses of a very strong, but very focused, magnetic field to parts of the brain. In depressive illness, the frontal regions of the brain are targeted. The TMS causes local inhibition of function (so, for example, if this is applied over the area of brain causing movement, a brief localised paralysis results). There is some published research indicating its effectiveness in depression, but more work is needed before it can be regarded as a reliable treatment. It does not seem, however, to hold out the hope of helping people with psychotic depression.

Should I take part in research programmes? My doctor has suggested that I might like to help with a trial of some new medication.

All prescribed medication has to be exhaustively tested, first in laboratories then on human volunteers. Without the people who have helped test medication, there would be no therapeutic drugs at all. So I'm in favour of all of us helping with scientific research, for the sake of each other. You will be thoroughly informed about exactly what you are taking, what possible side-effects there may be, and what benefits to expect. Your fully informed consent is necessary before you can be included in any clinical trials, and no one will expect you to take part in anything that you are not happy about.

What constitutes good scientific evidence for a treatment's benefits?

The gold standard is a double-blind, cross-over trial, comparing an active ingredient to a placebo (an inert substance) on two groups of carefully matched volunteer patients. 'Double-blind' means that neither the volunteer patient nor the doctor involved knows which people receive the active drug. 'Cross-over' means that the two groups of people swap treatments halfway through the trial, so that both groups have had the same intervention.

This can be quite difficult to do for some psychiatric treatments; how do you compare counselling with an inert substance, for example? How do you evaluate the effect of personal contact? So there are many other sorts of trial, and of course talking to our patients can teach us more than anything else.

How 'powerful' a trial is (that is, how much importance you can attach to its findings) will depend on how many people are involved in it. If the research is looking for a fairly rare occurrence, large numbers of people may be needed in the trial and 'control' groups to be sure that the difference in these groups has not merely arisen by chance.

The most powerful evidence comes from 'meta-analyses' where the results of a number of trials (which must have identical rules) can be added together.

Aren't there too many new drugs around for you to know the evidence about all of them?

A national body called 'NICE' (the National Institute for Clinical Excellence) has recently been formed to consider the evidence and form guidelines about new treatments, especially where a treatment is expensive or controversial. They publish guidelines on what is good practice.

The NHS has to be concerned not only with finding out what treatment works the best, but also with obtaining best value for money – the most cost-effective – so that our resources are not wasted on less effective treatments and so enabling more people to be treated. Most of NICE's work so far has been on expensive new treatments where there is some controversy, such as Aricept, the new treatment for Alzheimer's.

Bandolier is a fascinating medical journal published on the Internet, which is building up an ever increasing evidence base of good clinical trials. Currently there are more than 300 online journals participating. The Cochrane Collaboration is a group of enthusiasts who promote evidence-based medicine, and collect good quality clinical trial information.

Glossary

Words in *italics* have their own entry.

addiction A dependency on something that gives comfort. Usually refers to substances (legal or illegal), e.g. nicotine, alcohol, benzodiazepines, heroin, although the term is also used more loosely in connection with certain activities, e.g. gambling, overeating, workaholism, risk-taking, sexual behaviour – and even shopping. Addiction may be physical (involving your body) or psychological (involving the mind).

affective disorder A disturbance of emotion or mood. High, excited moods are found in manic states, and low moods are found in depressive illness. See also *bipolar disorder, depression, hypomania, mania, manic depression.*

Alzheimer's disease A progressive brain disorder, causing *Dementia.* This is commoner in old age and also in Down's syndrome. It causes shrinkage and degeneration of brain tissue. The effects are increasing loss of memory and reasoning ability. Whilst there is no known cure, recently introduced drugs such as Aricept may slow the deterioration.

analyst A *therapist* (customarily, but not always, a *psychiatrist*) who practises classical (psycho)analysis, as developed by Freud and his followers. Whilst this fascinating intellectual discipline was hugely influential in the birth of psychiatry and all the 'talking treatments', psychoanalysis plays little part nowadays in mainstream adult psychiatric treatment, not least because a course of analysis may take several years.

anorexia nervosa An eating disorder. Occurring mainly in adolescent girls (and less often in males), this consists of a distortion of body image so that the sufferer fears that she (or he) is unpleasantly fat. Despite all efforts at reassurance, the person will diet severely, losing over 15% of body weight and, in the case of females, periods will cease. *Bulimia nervosa* is a variation of anorexia. Both are serious and always warrant expert assessment.

antidepressant A class of drugs used to treat depression. Some types of antidepressants include tricyclics (*TCAs*), tetracyclics, monoamine oxidase inhibitors (*MAOIs*), selective serotonin re-uptake inhibitors (*SSRIs*), noradrenaline uptake reinhibitors (*NARIs*).

anxiety The natural response to any danger, threat or stress. Helps alert us to respond actively when under pressure; but, when it occurs out of context or in an exaggerated or disordered way, it can interfere with our daily lives. Anxiety frequently coexists with depression. See also *generalised anxiety disorder, obsessive compulsive disorder, panic disorder, post-traumatic stress disorder.*

Approved Social Worker (ASW) A social worker with training in dealing with mental illness. Will play a key part in *Section* procedures, as the person's representative.

art therapist Art therapy may be used in hospital or be provided as part of a *Community Mental Health Team's* resources. Drawing, painting, or other creative activities can be enjoyed at whatever level of ability. Sometimes it is easier to put emotion into paint or clay than into words, and quite a simple painting can be a real achievement. The work produced can be a powerful expression of feeling. Art therapists use art as a medium for therapy.

atypical antipsychotic drugs A group of drugs recently evolved to treat *psychotic* illnesses. Though more costly than older drugs, they may have fewer side-effects. Amisulpiride, clozapine, olanzepine, quetiapine, risperidone and zotepine are in this group.

benzodiazepine A family of minor tranquillisers. Includes Valium (diazepam), Librium (chlordiazepoxide), temazepam and nitrazepam. Effective for short-term reduction of anxiety, and as sleeping tablets. Because of their addictive potential, they are recommended *only* for short-term relief (2–4 weeks only) of severe, disabling or distressing anxiety or insomnia. Tolerance can even develop quicker than this, within 3–14 days of use. Withdrawal from long-term use has to be in gradual steps of perhaps one-eighth of the daily dose per fortnight. This may take from 4 weeks to 1 year.

bipolar affective disorder Also called *manic depressive illness*, bipolar disorder is a mood disorder in which spells of high excited mood (*hypomania* or *mania*) occur, as well as spells of *depression*. Mood-stabilising medication, including lithium and carbamazepine, helps prevent these episodes.

brain scan CT (computerised tomography) and MRI (magnetic resonance imaging) brain scans can be helpful in studying the structure of the brain and spinal cord, where injury or other disease may be present.

bulimia nervosa An eating disorder, involving food bingeing, then vomiting and purging, in which there are periods of feeling out of control with eating. Binges of large volumes of food occur, with attendant guilt and misery. These may be followed by vomiting and use of laxatives to try and limit the weight gained.

chronic fatigue syndrome A condition of 'severe, disabling fatigue, lasting at least 6 months, that affects both physical and mental functioning, and is present most of the time'. It may be triggered in a vulnerable person by a viral infection plus life stress, and it can lead to prolonged disability. Symptoms may include poor concentration, memory loss, sore lymph glands, muscle and joint pains, poor sleep, and exhaustion after exertion. Depression is often present. Evidence shows that prolonged rest is harmful. Graded exercise programmes and *cognitive behavioural therapy* have the highest success rates for treatment.

cognitive behaviour therapy A form of psychotherapy that concentrates on a person's current thoughts and feelings, and how we can alter the direct effects of them by practising more positive attitudes. Has been shown to be effective in various conditions including depression.

Community Psychiatric Nurse A psychiatric nurse who works outside hospital. May be attached to a GP surgery or to a Community Mental Health Team. He or she may keep in touch with a caseload of people with ongoing psychiatric problems, and some will also take on individual counselling.

counsellor Someone who provides counselling. May be based in a GP surgery, practise as an independent (private) practitioner, or be attached to a charitable organisation. The most experienced ones will have a qualification issued by the British Association of Counsellors and Psychotherapists (BACP).

craving An overwhelming desire; associated with addictions.

delusion A fixed, irrational belief. May be a part of a *psychosis*. Examples are feelings that one is being controlled by others or is being persecuted, that one has some dreadful illness, or is a famous person.

dementia A deteriorating illness causing loss of all mental functioning (memory, personality and thinking ability) caused by degeneration of the brain. *Alzheimer's disease* is one principal cause; repeated small strokes (multi-infarct dementia syndrome, MIDS) are another.

depot injection Some *neuroleptic* medication can be given in a slow release form, perhaps every 2–4 weeks, by deep intramuscular injection. This can be much more convenient than taking tablets daily. So far the newer, *atypical* drugs – with fewer side-effects – are not available in depot form.

discontinuation syndrome Some of the *SSRI antidepressant* drugs are associated with a group of symptoms that can occur when tablets are stopped or decreased suddenly. The symptoms can mimic anxiety. This does not mean that the illness is recurring but that the medication should be tailed off gradually, perhaps over 3–4 weeks.

dopamine A *neurotransmitter* that has an adrenaline-like action in the central nervous system.

drama therapy A form of psychotherapy that enables people to act out unspoken tensions and feelings, by playing through incidents or acting in roles, and having the content reflected back to them.

DSM4 The American Psychiatric Association has produced this national manual of definitions of psychiatric illness. See also *ICD10*.

ECT (electroconvulsive therapy) A treatment for certain types of severe depression. It involves inducing a carefully controlled seizure while the patient is deeply asleep under a brief general anaesthetic. It is highly effective and has saved many lives.

EEG (electroencephalogram) A recording made from electrodes applied to the scalp. It shows the levels of electrical activity in the brain and is helpful in diagnosing epilepsy, as well as other *organic illness.*

group therapy A powerful type of 'talking treatment'. In contrast to one-to-one therapy or counselling, groupwork involves a number of people meeting regularly and working together on a common problem. Strict rules about confidentiality are usually agreed upon ('What you hear here, stays here'). and a facilitator may be present to see fair play. Members of groups help support each other and find solutions from their own experiences to others' problems. Alcoholics Anonymous and Narcotics Anonymous, among others, use this format with good results.

hallucination A disturbance of one of the senses. A perception without a stimulus. May take the form of sights (e.g. visions), sounds (e.g. voices), touch, smells or tastes. Associated with psychotic illness, and can occur with both schizophrenic and bipolar disorders, as well as drug and alcohol misuse and withdrawal.

hypomania see under *Mania.*

ICD10 The International Classification of Disease is a classification of psychiatric illnesses. Produced by the World Health Organisation, it is designed to apply to every country in every major language. Like the DSM4, it can be used to help make a clear diagnosis from a group of symptoms, and also has information on some causes of illness.

lithium Lithium salts are used as mood stabilisers for bipolar – and sometimes unipolar – illness. It is also used in *resistant depression.* It is one of the few drugs that help prevent depressive illness. Blood tests are needed regularly.

mania A state of high excitement, with sleeplessness, flight of ideas, overactivity, and much mental energy and drive. *Delusions* and *hallucinations* can occur. Associated with *bipolar disorder.* The term *hypomania* is used for less severe forms of mania.

manic depression See *bipolar disorder.*

MAOI (monoamine oxidase inhibitor) A class of *antidepressant.* Early MAOIs had serious potential dietary interactions, and people taking these had to avoid certain foods, but the most recent version (moclobemide) is more user-friendly.

Mental Health Act 1983 This Act makes provision for the care of the psychiatrically ill. It defines when and how someone may be admitted to hospital under a compulsory order (known as a *'Section'* procedure).

MIDS (multi-infarct dementia syndrome) A cause of dementia, following a series of small strokes. See also *Alzheimer's disease*.

NARI (noradrenaline re-uptake inhibitor) A class of *anti-depressants* that acts by reducing the rate at which noradrenaline is removed from the *synapse*.

neuroleptics Drugs used to treat psychotic illnesses. Also helpful with extreme anxiety states, and especially useful because they are not habit forming.

neurology The study of diseases of the nervous system.

neuropharmacology The study of drugs that affect the brain and nervous system.

neurophysiology The study of nervous system functioning. This includes the study of EEGs, nerve conduction and muscle studies.

neuropsychiatry The branch of medicine that spans psychiatry and neurology.

neurosis A group of mental illnesses, where contact is kept with reality. Examples are neurotic depression, anxiety, phobias and obsessional states. Sufferers experience normal emotions but in an exaggerated, inappropriate, even disabling, way, causing disruption and reduced levels of functioning. Unfortunately the term 'neurotic' has been devalued and has become insulting in general parlance.

neurotransmitter Chemicals that act between the ends of the nerve cells of the brain and spinal column to send messages – either to stimulate or to reduce activity – to different organs: nerves, muscles or glandular structures. Acetylcholine, dopamine, serotonin, adrenaline, GABA and noradrenaline are some of the main types. *Antidepressants* act by altering their levels, i.e. by inhibiting their re-uptake (as do the *SSRIs*) or by reducing their breakdown rates (as do the *MAOIs*).

noradrenaline One of the key *neurotransmitters*.

organic illness A mental disturbance caused by a recognisable disease process. Conditions such as uncontrolled diabetes, severe urinary or chest infections, liver failure, head injury, epilepsy and drug withdrawal can all cause mental disturbances.

panic disorder A form of anxiety, where the sufferer suddenly experiences overwhelming anxiety and may feel that they are dying.

These panic attacks can occur on a background of continuing *anxiety*. Palpitations (fast heartbeat), sweating and overbreathing can occur. Relaxation training, *CBT*, and *antidepressant* treatment are all effective.

paranoia A form of *delusion*, involving feelings of persecution or jealousy. May be part of a *psychosis*. The term 'paranoid personality' is used to describe a sensitive, suspicious personality type.

Parkinson's disease Caused by damage to *dopamine*-producing cells in a specific area of the brain, Parkinson's disease causes a progressively stiff, slow, shuffling gait, with a 'pill-rolling' tremor of the hands, tiny handwriting, and a featureless, unsmiling face. Treatment is by increasing *dopamine* levels with drugs such as levodopa. It is associated with mood disorders, and can sometimes be associated with dementia.

phobia An excessive, irrational fear of some specific object or situation.

psychiatrist A medically trained doctor who has a special interest and further training in psychiatric illnesses and in dealing with emotional and behavioural disorders.

psychoanalyst A therapist who practises classical analysis. Based on Freud's theory, this can consist of regular sessions over several years. Although the traditional image of the psychiatrist includes the patient lying on Freud's couch, analysis is no longer part of mainstream psychiatric treatment.

psychologist A university graduate with a degree in the study of behaviour and its mental processes. Clinical psychologists are often part of hospital or community mental health teams. They may evaluate memory, intelligence, personality and emotions. Other branches of psychology include educational and industrial psychology.

psychosis A mental illness in which there is a loss of contact with reality, delusions, and an inability to see this as illness. There may also be hallucinations. Psychosis may be produced by many different causes: very severe depression, part of some physical illness, *bipolar disorder, schizophrenia, schizoaffective disorder*, and drug or alcohol abuse.

psychotherapist Someone who carries out talking therapy; or any of the many types of psychotherapy. These include cognitive behavioural therapy and interpersonal therapy.

PTSD (post-traumatic stress disorder) Exposure to a severe trauma outside normal experience, which would cause suffering in almost everybody. It causes intense fear and helplessness, with nightmares and flashbacks, sometimes triggered later by less serious upsets. It leads to overarousal and sleep disturbance, with avoidance of situations that recall the trauma. Sufferers may overuse alcohol, making symptoms worse.

PubMed This is a World Wide Web (WWW) retrieval service developed by the US National Library of Medicine. It provides access, free of charge, to MEDLINE, a database of more than 10 million health-related scientific publications. PubMed is an easy-to-use search tool for finding medical research articles that have been published in peer-reviewed journals (i.e. scrutinised by experts). Users search by entering a few key words or phrases. Search on ncbi.nlm.nih.gov/PubMed/

resistant depression Depression which fails to respond to two courses of at least 8 weeks of full doses of antidepressants taken regularly. Management may involve combinations of treatments, e.g. CBT plus medication and addressing possible triggers.

RIMA (reversible inhibition of monoamine oxidase inhibitor) A recently developed *MAOI*. This *antidepressant* has fewer food and drug interactions than the original versions.

Royal College of Psychiatrists The academic institution that sets national standards for psychiatric training. Entrance is by examination, and members will have the letters MRCPsych after their name. This qualification enables a doctor to follow a career in psychiatry. The College publishes two journals, the *Psychiatric Bulletin* and the *British Journal of Psychiatry*. These are accessible via *PubMed*.

schizoaffective disorder This illness involves a mixture of mood disorder plus some symptoms of schizophrenia; it has a better outcome than the latter condition.

schizophrenia This psychotic illness affects about 1% of the population. It varies in its severity and form. It is characterised by delusions, hallucinations (most often auditory or 'voices') and ideas of being controlled in mind or body.

seasonal affective disorder (SAD) Low moods associated with low levels of sunlight, e.g. during winter months. Light therapy may be helpful.

'Section' procedure A compulsory admission procedure under the *Mental Health Act*. Usually involves two doctors, and an *Approved Social Worker (ASW)*. Can only be used where a patient is a risk to their own health or to that of someone else, owing to a mental illness.

Section 12 Doctor A doctor with experience in the diagnosis and management of mental illness, who is approved to take part in compulsory admission procedures under the *Mental Health Act*.

sedation Relaxing or calming someone who is distressed or agitated, e.g. with medication.

serotonin One of the brain's main *neurotransmitter* chemicals. Low levels of serotonin are associated with depression. *SSRI* drugs work as antidepressants by increasing brain levels of serotonin.

social phobia A form of anxiety disorder, involving extreme shyness, and intense difficulty with being among other people. This condition may be quite disabling, and can lead to heavy alcohol use. Treatment with cognitive behaviour therapy and SSRIs is effective.

SSRI (selective serotonin re-uptake inhibitor) A newer class of antidepressants. Safe in overdose, and has fewer contraindications and side effects than older antidepressants (TCAs, MAOIs), although more expensive.

stress Any change (whether physical, psychological or social, welcome or unwelcome) that requires us to adapt. Responses to stress may be useful or unhelpful, even damaging. Life without some stress would be unimaginable.

synapse The gap at the end of a nerve cell, through which *neurotransmitters* travel, sending impulses to other nerves, muscle or gland tissue. This is the site at which *antidepressants* act.

syndrome A collection of symptoms, which together are characteristic of a particular illness.

TCAs (tricyclic antidepressants) These older drugs are as effective as any newer ones, but have different interactions or contraindications. For example, they should be used with caution if a patient has heart disease or glaucoma.

tolerance The dose of certain drugs needs to be increased to obtain the same effect as time goes by. For example, the dose of sleeping tablets, such as the benzodiazepines, may need to be increased as their effect wears off.

tranquilliser (major and minor) Medication that calms or relaxes. 'Minor' tranquillisers may be helpful for anxiety and insomnia, and include the benzodiazepines. 'Major' tranquillisers (more often known as neuroleptics) are helpful in anxiety and also psychotic illness.

withdrawal symptoms Unpleasant feelings when you have to go without a particular substance. May be psychological (anxiety, irritability and poor sleep) or physical (restlessness, sweats, muscle cramps). Some substances, e.g. alcohol and benzodiazepines, can trigger fits if heavy users stop suddenly. Symptoms vary with the substance: Valium withdrawal, for example, may last over several weeks and symptoms include restlessness, broken sleep, anxiety, nightmares and, in severe cases, fits. *Antidepressants* do not cause withdrawal but some *SSRIs* need to be tailed off gradually to avoid a *discontinuation syndrome*.

Appendix 1
Useful addresses and websites

If there is no other indication, websites begin with www.

General

Age Concern England
Astral House
1268 London Road
London SW16 4ER
Helpline: 0800 009966
Tel: (020) 8679 8000
Fax: (0208) 766 7211
Website: ace.org.uk
Researches into the needs of older people and is involved in policy making. Publishes many books and has useful fact sheets on a wide range of issues from benefits to care, and provides services via local branches.

Association for Postnatal Illness (APNI)
145 Dawes Road
London SW6 7EB
Tel: (0207) 386 0868
Fax: (0207) 386 8885
Website: apni.org
Help and advice for sufferers and families affected by postnatal illness. Network of local contacts.

AWARE – Helping to defeat depression
72 Lower Leeson Street
Dublin 2
Ireland
Helpline: 00 353 1 676 6166 (10 am–10 pm 7 days a week) (from UK)
Tel: 00 353 1 661 7208 (from UK)
Fax: 00 353 1 661 7217
Website: aware.ie
Offers support and information to sufferers and families affected by depression. Funds research into its causes.

British Epilepsy Association
New Anstey House
Gateway Drive
Yeadon
Leeds LS19 7XI
Helpline: 08808 800 5050
Tel: (0113) 210 8800
Fax: (0113) 391 0300
Website: epilepsy.org.uk
Provides help, information and advice for everyone with epilepsy, their families and carers. Literature, self-help groups, specialist nurses and insurance also available.

Calm
Helpline: 0800 585858
A Helpline for young men who are depressed or suicidal.

Carers National Association
20–25 Glasshouse Yard
London EC1A 4JT
Helpline: 0808 808 7777
Tel: (0207) 490 8818
Fax: (0207) 490 8824
Website: carers.demon.co.uk
Offers information and support to all people who have to care for others due to medical or other problems.

Contact a Family
209–211 City Road
London EC1V 1JN
Helpline: 0808 808 3555
Tel: (0207) 608 8701
Fax: (0207) 608 8701
Website: cafamily.org.uk
Offers helpline for parents of children with special needs. Also has comprehensive information of rare syndromes affecting people of all ages. Looseleaf directory also available.

Cruse Bereavement Care
Cruse House
126 Sheen Road
Richmond TW9 1UR
Helpline: 0870 167 1677
Tel: (0208) 940 4818
Fax: (0208) 940 7638
Website:
crusebereavementcare.org.uk
Offers information and literature and has local branches that can provide 1 to 1 counselling. Training in bereavement for professionals.

Department of Work and Pensions
Disability Benefit Centre
Olympic House
Olympic Way
Wembley HA9 0DL
Helpline: 0800 88 22 00
Tel: (0208) 795 8400
Government information service offering advice on benefits for people with disabilities and their carers.

Depression Alliance
35 Westminster Bridge Road
London SE1 7JB
Tel: (0207) 633 9929
Fax: (0207) 633 0559
Website: depressionalliance.org.uk
Information, support and understanding for people who suffer with depression and for relatives who want help. Produces a series of leaflets including Depression, Can't face the world, *and* Depression and your sex life. *Has a network of self-help groups and correspondence schemes. Send SAE for information.*

Families Anonymous
Doddington and Rollo Community
Association
Charlotte Despard Avenue
Battersea
London SW11 5JE
Tel: (0207) 498 4680
Fax: (0207) 498 1990
Website: faminon.org.uk
Community association that sells literature, offers telephone support and refers to other agencies as appropriate. Has local support group.

Fellowship of Depressives Anonymous
PO Box FDA
Self-help, Nottingham
Ormiston House
32–36 Pelham Street
Nottingham NG1 2EG
Tel: (01702) 433838
Fax: (01702) 433843
Organisation run as a source of support for sufferers from depression, complementary to professional care.

Meet a Mum Association
Waterside Centre
25 Avenue Road
London SE25 4DX
Helpline: (0208) 768 0123
Tel: (0208) 771 5595
Website: mama.org.uk
An organisation offering support to women suffering from postnatal depression.

Men Against Violence
Tel: (01438) 747074
This is local group in Hertfordshire, but it has a national telephone helpline used through referral by probation officers and police. Men's groups such as this may be available in your area. Try contacting NHS Direct, your local Citizens' Advice Bureau or the telephone book.

Mental Health Drugs
Maudsley Hospital
Denmark Hill
London SE5 8AZ
Helpline: (0207) 919 2999
Tel: (0207) 919 2317
Medicines information helpline run by pharmacists at the Maudsley Hospital for patients and carers from 11 am to 5 pm. The second Telline offers advice to health professionals from 9 am to 5.30 pm.

Mental Health Foundation
20/21 Cornwall Terrace
London NW1 4QL
Tel: (0207) 535 7400
Fax: (0207) 535 7474
Website: mentalhealth.org.uk
A major UK charity working with mental health and learning disability. Offers information and publications, gives grants for research and community projects related to mental health welfare. Contributes to public debate and influencing policy makers and health care professionals.

MIND (National Association for Mental Health)
Granta House
15–19 Broadway
London E15 4BQ
Helpline: 0845 766 0163
Tel: (0208) 519 2122
Fax: (0208) 522 1725
Website: mind.org.uk
Mental health organisation working for a better life for everyone experiencing mental distress. Has information and offers support via local branches.

National Association for Premenstrual Syndrome (NAPS)
7 Swift's Court
High Street
Seal
Sevenoaks TN15 0EG
Tel/Fax: (01732) 760011
Website: pms.org.uk
The NAPS exists for women suffering from PMS; it is staffed by professionals and fellow sufferers. There is also a helpline offering advice to partners of PMS sufferers. Their database gathers information on latest research developments.

National Childbirth Trust
Alexandra House
Oldham Terrace
Acton
London W3 6NH
Helpline: 08704 448708
Tel: 08704 448707
Fax: 08707 703237
Website:
nctpregnancyandbabycare.com
Parent-to-parent support via local groups. Antenatal classes and breastfeeding counselling by trained teachers. Breastfeeding counselling helpline available 8 am to 10 pm.

National Debtline
Birmingham Settlement
318 Summer Lane
Birmingham B19 3RL
Helpline: 0808 808 4000
Tel: 08459 500511
Fax: (0121) 248 3070
Website:
birminghamsettlement.org.uk
Offers information and advice on debts relating to mortgages and rent; how to work out a personal budget, negotiate with creditors and deal with court procedures.

NHS Direct
Tel: 0845 4647 or 0800 665544 (if you do not have an NHS Direct yet in your area)
NHS helpline staffed by qualified nurses who give medical advice on all aspects of health over the telephone and refer to local hospitals in emergencies.

Patients Association
PO Box 935
Harrow HA1 3YJ
Helpline: 0845 608 4455
Tel: (0208) 423 9111
Fax: (0208) 423 9119
Website: patients-association.com
Provides advice on patients' rights. 'Patients are the reason for the NHS not interruptions to it.' A campaigning organisation working on behalf of patients.

The Pre-Retirement Association
9 Chesham Road
Guildford GU1 3LS
Tel: (01483) 301170
Fax: (01483) 300981
Website: pra.uk.com
Runs courses and produces literature on the subject of retirement for employees and employers. Produces a newsletter dedicated to mid-life and retirement planning.

Relate (National Marriage Guidance)
Herbert Gray College
Little Church Street
Rugby CV21 3AP
Helpline: 09069 123715
Tel: (01788) 573241
Fax: (01788) 535007
Website: relate.org.uk
Offers relationship counselling via local branches and publications from Relate bookshop including mailorder. Will discuss health, sexual, self-esteem, depression, bereavement, remarriage issues.

Release
Helpline: (0207) 603 8654
Tel: (0207) 729 9904
Offers information over the telephone on legal and illegal drugs.

Royal College of Psychiatrists
17 Belgrave Square
London SW1X 8PG
Tel: (0207) 235 2351
Fax: (0207) 245 1231
Website: rcpsych.ac.uk
Professional body holding lists of qualified psychiatrists. Patients must be referred by GPs.

Samaritans
10 The Grove
Slough SL1 1QP
Helpline: 08745 909090
Tel: (01753) 216500
Fax: (01753) 819004
Website: samaritans.org.uk
National organisation offering confidential support to those in distress who feel suicidal or despairing and need someone to talk to. The Samaritans have 204 branches around the country open 24 hours a day, every day of the year. The telephone number of your local branch can be found in the telephone directory. Most branches also see visitors at certain times of the day: phone the local branch for information. You will get a reply to an email within 24 hours.

SANE
1st Floor Cityside House
40 Adler Street
London E1 1EE
SANELINE: 0345 678000
Helpline: 0845 767 8000
Tel: (0207) 375 1002
Fax: (0207) 375 2162
Website: sane.org.uk
A mental charity that runs a helpline offering emotional and crisis support to people with mental health problems, their families and friends. It funds research into mental illness and gives access to extensive literature including information for professionals and organisations working in the field. Has a database of local and national services.

SCOPE (formerly the Spastics Society)
6 Market Road
London N7 9PW
Helpline: 0808 800 3333
Tel: (0207) 619 7100
Fax: (0207) 619 7399
Website: scope.org.uk
Provides information and counselling service on cerebral palsy and associated disabilities. It manages a number of schools, education centres, units and residential centres for people with cerebral palsy.

Seasonal Affective Disorder Association (SADA)
PO Box 989
Steyning BN44 3HG
Website: sada.org.uk
Offers support and information on seasonal affective disorder and details of light therapy and equipment. Local support groups have a lightbox hire scheme. Enquiries by letter welcomed; SAE requested.

Social Services Benefits
Helpline: 0800 882200

Threshold
Womens Mental Health Information Line
14 St Georges Place
Brighton BN1 4GB
Helpline: (01273) 626 444
Tel: 0845 300 0911
Fax: (01273) 626444
National information line on mental health for men and women. Also offers local referrals in the Brighton area.

Victim Support Scheme
National Office
Cranmer House
39 Brixton Road
London SW9 6DZ
Helpline: 0845 303 0900
Tel: (0207) 735 9166
Fax: (0207) 582 5712
Website: victimsupport.com
Offers emotional support and practical advice through local support groups to people who have been victims of crime.

Women's Aid
PO Box 391
Bristol BS99 7WS
Helpline: 08457 023 468
Tel: (0117) 944 4411
Fax: (0117) 924 1703
Website: womensaid.org.uk
Runs a national helpline for advice, information and refuge referrals for women and children experiencing domestic violence.

Women's Health
52 Featherstone Street
London
EC1Y 8RT
Helpline: (020) 490 5489
Tel: (020) 7251 6580
Fax: (020) 7250 4152
Website: womenshealthlondon.org.uk
*Provides information to help women
make informed decisions about
their health, and a range of
publications and quarterly
newsletter. To use reference library,
telephone first.*

Workaholics Anonymous
PO Box 11466
London SW1V 2ZQ
*Contact by post only. Workaholics
Anonymous is a small self-help
group patterned after Alcoholics
Anonymous. Information will be
sent to all enquirers.*

Alcohol and drug abuse problems

Al-Anon Family Groups
61 Great Dover Street
London SE1 4YF
Tel: (0207) 403 0888
Fax: (0207) 378 9910
Website: hexnet.co.uk/alanon/
*Offers support to families and
friends of problem drinkers; can
refer to local groups. Alateen is
dedicated to helping children aged
12 to 20 with an alcoholic relative.*

Alcoholics Anonymous (AA)
Baltic Chambers
50 Wellington Street
Glasgow G2 6HJ
Helpline: 0845 769 7555
Tel: (0141) 226 2214
Website:
alcoholics-anonymous.org.uk
and
PO Box 1
Stonebow House
Stonebow
York YO1 7NJ
Tel: (01904) 644 026
*Offers information and support, via
local groups, to people with an
alcohol problem who want to stop
drinking.*

**Council for Involuntary
Tranquilliser Addiction (CITA)**
Cavendish House
Brighton Road
Waterloo
Liverpool L22 5NG
Helpline: (0151) 949 0102
Tel: (0151) 474 9626
Fax: (0151) 284 8324
*Offers information on tranquilliser
addition and a helpline with
specialist counsellors.*

Drinkline (National Alcohol Helpline)
1st Floor
Cavern Court
8 Mathew Street
Liverpool L2 6RE
Helpline: 0800 917 8282
Asian Line: 0990 133481 – in Hindi, Urdu, Gujerati, Punjabi
Tel: (0151) 227 4150
Fax: (0151) 227 4019
Website: wrecked.co.uk
Funded by Dept. of Health, Drinkline provides information and self-help materials to those concerned about their drinking habits and friends and relatives. Refer to local agencies for support.

Drugs in Schools
Helpline: 0808 8000 800
Website: schoolchoice.co.uk/ad.info/a_art/release.art.html

Institute for the Study of Drug Dependence (ISDD)
Waterbridge House
32–36 Loman Street
London SE1 0EE

Narcotics Anonymous (NA)
Helpline: (0207) 730 0009
Voluntary organisation offering information on drugs and support over the telephone and at meetings.

National Drugs Helpline
Tel: 0800 776600

Quit
Victory House
170 Tottenham Court Road
London W1P 0HA
Tel: 0800 002200

Release
388 Old Street
London EC1V 9LY
Tel: (0207) 729 9904/603 8654
Website: drugshouse.org.uk/helplines.html

Standing Conference on Drug Abuse
Waterbridge House
32–36 Loman Street
London SE1 0EE
Tel: (0207) 928 9500

Alternative therapy

British Acupuncture Council
63 Jeddo Road
London W12 9HQ
Tel: (0208) 735 0400
Fax: (0208) 735 0404
Website: acupuncture.org.uk
Professional body offering lists of qualified acupuncture therapists.

British Herbal Medicine Association
Sun House
Church Street
Stroud GL5 1SL
Tel: (01453) 751389
Fax: (01453) 751402
Provides lists of qualified herbalists, offers information service on products and legalities for importers and vets advertisements.

British Medical Acupuncture Society
12 Marbury House
Higher Whitley
Warrington WA4 4QW
Tel: (01925) 730727
Fax: (01925) 730492
Website: medical_acupuncture.co.uk
Professional body offering training to doctors and list of accredited practitioners.

Institute for Complementary Medicine
PO Box 194
London SE16 1QZ
Tel: (0207) 237 5165
Fax: (0207) 237 5175
Website: icmedicine.co.uk
Umbrella group for complementary medicine organisations.

Anxiety states

Anxiety Care
Cardinal Heenan Centre
326 High Road
Ilford IG1 1QP
Helpline: (0208) 478 3400
Tel: (0208) 262 8891
Fax: (0208) 262 8680
Website: anxietycare.org.uk
Offer information and support as well as 1 to 1 counselling for people with anxiety disorders.

First Steps to Freedom
7 Avon Court
School Lane
Kenilworth CV8 2GX
Tel: (01926) 851608
Fax: 0870 164 0567
Website: firststeps.demon.co.uk

National Phobics Society
Zion Community Resource Centre
339 Stretford Road
Hulme
Manchester M15 4ZY
Tel: 0870 770 0456
Tel: (0161) 227 9898
Fax: (0161) 227 9862
Website: phobics-society.org.uk
Provides information and support groups and can refer to trained hypnotherapists.

No Panic (National Organisation for Phobias, Anxiety, Neuroses Information and Care)
93 Brands Farm Way
Randlay
Telford TF3 2JQ
Recorded information line:
0800 783 1531
Helpline: (01952) 590545
(10 am–10 pm every day)
A self-help group for people with obsessive compulsive disorders.

Obsessive Action
Aberdeen Centre
22–24 Highbury Grove
London N5 2EA
Tel: (0207) 226 4000
Fax: (0207) 288 0828
Website: obsessive-action.demon.co.uk/index.htm

Triumph Over Phobia (Top UK)
PO Box 1831
Bath BA2 4YW
Tel: (01225) 330353
Fax: (01225) 469212
Website: triumphoverphobia.com
*Has network of self-help groups
offering information and support
for people affected by obsessive
compulsive disorders.*

Children

Childline
Helpline: 0800 1111
Tel: (0207) 239 1000
Fax: (0207) 239 1001
Website: childline.org.uk
*Confidential support and advice
phoneline for young people with
problems of any kind. They offer
counselling and referral to
appropriate agencies. Outreach
visits to schools and information
sheets.*

Off the Record
Open House Centre
Manvers Street
Bath BA1 1JW
Helpline: 0800 389 5551
Tel/Fax: (01225) 312481
Website: offtherecord-banes.co.uk
*A free and confidential young
peoples advice and counselling
service. Has a drop-in centre and
offers special projects for young
carers and homeless youngsters in
the Bath area. Also helps young
parents and professionals. Visits
schools.*

Parentline
Helpline: 0808 800 2222 (9 am–9 pm
Mon–Thurs)
Helpline and information for parents
in distress

Young Minds Trust
The Children's Mental Health Charity
102–108 Clerkenwell Road
London EC1M 5SA
Helpline: 0800 018 2138 10 am–1 pm
Mon/Fri; 9 am–4 pm Tue–Thurs)
Tel: (0207) 336 8445
Fax: (0207) 336 8446
Website: youngminds.org.uk
*Offers an information service to
parents, consultancy, seminars and
training. Also has leaflets and
booklets for young people.*

Youth Access
1 & 2 Taylors Yard
67 AldebrookRoad
London SW12 8AD
Tel: (0208) 772 9900
Fax: (0208) 772 9746
*This umbrella organisation can give
sources of information, advice and
counselling for young people in all
areas. When not attended,
answerphone message refers callers
to Childline and Samaritans.*

Counselling/
psychotherapy

**Association of Women
Psychotherapists**
Tel: (0208) 202 0816

British Association for Behavioural and Cognitive Psychotherapies
PO Box 9
Accrington BB5 2GD
Tel/Fax: (01254) 875277
Website: babcp.org
Can provide a directory of registered therapists for a small fee.

British Association for Counselling and Psychotherapy
1 Regent Place
Rugby CV21 2PJ
Tel: 08788 550899
Fax: 0870 443 5161
Website: counselling.co.uk
Professional services organisation and impartial register for counsellors. Offers lists of all levels of counsellors and can refer to specialist counselling services.

British Association of Psychotherapists
37 Mapesbury Road
London NW2 4HJ
Tel: (0208) 452 9823
Fax: (0208) 452 5182
Website: bap-psychotherapy.org.uk

British Confederation of Psychotherapists
37 Mapesbury Road
London NW2 4HJ
Tel: (0208) 830 5173
Fax: (0208) 452 3684
Website: bcp.org.uk
Professional umbrella body for psychotherapists who cover psycho-analytic psychotherapy and child psychosis. Have list of qualified therapists.

British Psychological Society
St Andrews House
48 Princess Road East
Leicester LE1 7DR
Tel: (0116) 254 9568
Fax: (0116) 247 0787
Website: bps.org.uk
Provides national list of accredited psychologists on receipt of SAE.

PACE
Tel: 0207) 697 0017 (10 am–9 pm Mon–Thurs)
Counselling, mental health advocacy and group work for lesbians and gay men.

UK Council for Psychotherapy (UKCP)
167–169 Great Portland Street
London W1W 5PF
Tel: (0207) 436 3002
Fax: (0207) 436 3013
Website: psychotherapy.org.uk
Regulatory body and impartial organisation for psychotherapists. Maintains national register of therapists and information on training.

UK Register of Counsellors
PO Box 1050
Rugby CV21 2HZ
Tel: 0870 443 5232
Fax: 0870 443 5161
Part of the British Association of Counselling and Psychotherapy. Regulatory body which provides details of registered counsellors offering safe and accountable practice.

Eating problems

Eating Disorders Association
1st Floor Wensum House
103 Prince of Wales Place
Norwich NR1 1DW
Helpline: (01603) 621 414
Youthline: (01603) 765050
Tel: (01603) 619 090
Fax: (01603) 664 915
Website: edauk.com
*Offers information, help and
support to anyone affected by eating
disorders – anorexia and bulimia
nervosa. Local self-help groups.*

Overeaters Anonymous
OA-GB
PO Box 19
Stratford
Manchester M32 9EB
Helpline: 07000 784985
Tel: (01603) 259173
Website: oagb.org
*Offers support and recovery from a
variety of disorders: obesity,
compulsive eating, bulimia and
anorexia via meetings, telephone,
letters and working the 12 Steps to
Freedom, similar to Alcoholic
Anonymous.*

Manic depression

Manic Depression Fellowship
Castle Works
21 St Georges Road
London SE1 6ES
Tel: (0207) 793 2600
Fax: (0207) 793 2639
Website: mdf.org.uk
*Offers information and training to
people affected by manic depression.
Has local support groups that offer
self-management training.*

Internet news groups

If you are Internet proficient, try
searching for:

alt.support.depression

alt.support.phobias

sci.psychology

sci.med

sci.med.psychobiology

Websites

These spring up like mushrooms, and
some caution is advised when
looking for websites, as they can be
sponsored by all sorts of people.

**ability.org/Obsessive_
Compulsive_Disorder.html**
*This website is aimed at people with
(dis)abilities. It contains a wide
range of mental health information.*

**anxietycare.org/documents/
OCD-causesonline.htm**
Based in east London, this charity
helps people to recover from anxiety
disorders and to stay well. It has
email (see above addresses) and
online chat rooms.

depressionalliance.org.uk
This charity organisation is run by,
and for, people with depression. The
website contains information about
symptoms, treatments, campaigns,
penfriends, and local self-help
groups.

familyinternet.com/quackwatch
A famous American site aimed at
combating health-related fraud,
myths, fads, fallacies and quackery!

jr2.ox.ac.uk/Bandolier/index/htm
Voted the best website in 1999,
Bandolier collects, distils and
presents the best evidence about
treatments for doctors and patients
alike, using systematic reviews.
Contains some mental health
information.

iop.kcl.ac.uk/main/Mhealth
The Maudsley page. Produced by the
Institute of Psychiatry and the
South London/ Maudsley Trust, this
site has a good mental health page
for adult and childhood illnesses, as
well as detailed information about
research and teaching. It contains
information about the Maudsley
Family Study on manic depression,
a national survey of this condition.

mentalhealth.com
Another American site, which could
also be of interest to UK surfers.
Clear information on a wide range
of mental health conditions.

nhsdirect.nhs.uk
Besides giving telephone advice on
all health matters NHS Direct has a
large comprehensive health website
on which you can search for information and advice about many
medical conditions. There are useful
links to a wide range of publications, self-help organisations and
other resources. There is a good link
for a site on depression commis-
sioned by NHS Direct Online from
the Centre of Evidence-Based Mental
Health at Oxford University. The
site includes: What is depression?
How is depression diagnosed? How
is it treated? Overcoming depression; Lifestyle and depression, and
includes clips of someone talking
about their experience of this illness
and a wide range of information
about diet and self-help.

ocdhelp.org/faq.html
An international (though US-based)
organisation with 10,000 members
– for people with Obsessive
Compulsive Disorder, and their
family, friends and carers.

Pendulum is a mailing list for people diagnosed with bipolar mood disorder (manic depression) and related disorders and their supporters, and some professionals. To subscribe to Pendulum, send a message to majordomo@ncar.ucar.edu containing the line: subscribe pendulum

ppphealthcare.co.uk
This private healthcare website has some useful information on common mental health problems.

primhe.org
Primary Care Mental Health Education is an association for professionals interested in primary care mental health.

sandwellmind.co.uk
This website is a bookshop, associated with Amazon, which lists many books on Mental Health.

vh.org
'Virtual Hospital' and 'Virtual Children's Hospital' are US internet sites for doctors and patients, containing a wide and fascinating range of health information. Some good mental health topics are included.

youngminds.org.uk
YoungMinds is a national children's mental health charity. Its services include a parents' Information Service and Helpline (0800 018 2138

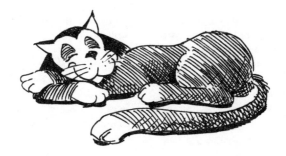

Appendix 2
Useful publications
and Internet information

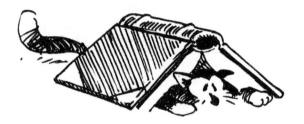

The AA member – medications & other drugs. Available from Alcoholics Anonymous (0845 769 7555).

The addictive personality, by Craig Nakken, Hazeldon Publications, 1996. This book is relevant to anyone who uses addictions of any kind to cope.

All in the end is the harvest, edited by Agnes Whitaker, DLT, 1984. An anthology for anyone who is grieving.

The anatomy of melancholy, by Robert Burton, 1620. One of the earliest books to tackle this subject. A great literary classic.

The anxiety and phobia workbook, by Edmund Bourne, New Harbinger Publications, 2001.

Coping with chronic fatigue, by Trudie Chalder, Sheldon Press, 1995. A very good self-help book for anyone suffering from chronic fatigue from whatever cause.

Getting better bit(e) by bit(e), by Schmidt and Treasure, Lawrence Erlbaum Assoc. Publications, 1993. Reprinted 1999. A good and helpful self-help guide for people with eating disorders.

Living in fear, by Isaac Marks, McGraw Hill, 2001. A clear and practical self-help book for anyone coping with anxiety and phobias.

The NCT book of postnatal depression, by Heather Welford, HarperCollins, 1998.

The noonday demon: an atlas of depression, by Andrew Solomon, Chatto & Windus, 2001.An informed and compassionate book about the history of depression, and the author's own battles with it.

The scent of dried roses, by Tim Lott, Penguin, 1997. A moving account of his, and his mother's, major depressive illnesses, and how society's attitude to depression has changed in recent years.

So sad, so young, so listen, by Philip Graham and Carol Hughes, Royal College of Psychiatrists, 1995. An excellent booklet about depression in children and teenagers, for parents, teachers, and children themselves.

A special scar, by Alison Wertheimer, Routledge, 2001. This book looks at the stigma surrounding suicide and offers practical help for survivors, relatives and friends of people who have taken their own life. Fifty

bereaved people tell their own stories. They show how they have learnt to live with the suicide, offering hope to others facing this 'personal holocaust'.

Staying sane, by Raj Persaud, Bantam, 2001.

Stop blaming, start loving, by Bill O'Hanlon and Pat Hudson, WW Norton & Co., 1996. A solution-orientated approach to improving your relationship.

Surviving postnatal depresssion, by Cara Aiken, Jessica Kingsley Publishers, 2000.

Touched with fire; manic-depressive illness and the artistic temperament, by Kay Redfield Jamison, The Free Press (Macmillan), New York, 1993. The author , who herself has manic depressive illness, discusses the lives of some great artists and how their creativity related to this condition.

A woman in your own right, by Anne Dickson, Quartet Publications, 1982. Reprinted 1999. A clear and helpful book on assertiveness for women.

Women who love too much, by Robin Norwood, Arrow Publications, 1986. This is a very helpful book for any woman in an abusive relationship.

Chatrooms and forums on the Internet

Chatrooms can be helpful as a way of talking to other people with problems that may be similar to your own, although, in some of the whackier ones, some people seem to use them as an outlet for their anger and distress, which may make upsetting reading for everyone else.

A patient of mine described one particular chatroom as 'like reading the graffiti in a public toilet'. So be careful as an unpleasant remark on the Internet can be pretty distressing; it's all too easy to type in some bad stuff and hit the send button. Never, ever, arrange to meet people from chatrooms.

Bandolier – see the Websites above.

Leaflets

Information on the following leaflets is from the NHS Direct website.

About Depression Alliance
Describes different types of depression, suggests various measures of self-help and gives details about drug and talking treatments available. The last section gives information about the Depression Alliance, which aims to establish a self-help group in every town.
Contact Depression Alliance (see Appendix 1).

All about depression
Written for people who may have depression, their friends or family, it explains the nature of depression, how it may affect different people and the various types of treatment, such as drug therapy, talking treatments and self-help, as well as hospital treatments. It has details about other self-help groups and references for further reading about depression.
Contact Mental Health Foundation (see Appendix 1).

Depression & antidepressants
Looks at commonly used antidepressants and details different types of antidepressants, how they work, possible side-effects, when they are safe to take and possible special precautions.
Contact Depression Alliance (see Appendix 1).

Postnatal depression
Describes how a woman may experience depression after the birth of a child including baby blues, depression and puerperal psychosis. It gives information to help the reader recognise each condition and advice about alleviating the symptoms. It includes references for further reading and details about support groups.
Contact the National Childbirth Trust (see Appendix 1).

Understanding depression
Published in association with the BMA, this booklet describes the nature of depression and its possible causes. It suggests self-help methods, and gives details of treatments and medication. There is advice for friends and family, contact details for many support groups and references for further reading.
Published by Family Doctor Publications Ltd, 10 Butchers Row, Banbury, Oxon, OX16 8JH. Tel: (01295) 276627; Fax: (01295) 276626.

Understanding depression
Explains what depression is, the symptoms and causes, and gives details about the treatments available. These include talking treatments (for instance counselling, cognitive behaviour therapy and psychotherapy), drugs, hospital admission, electroconvulsive therapy (ECT), and alternative therapies. There is a section giving advice to friends and relatives and a list of useful organisations and other publications.
Contact Mind (see Appendix 1).

Understanding postnatal depression
Postnatal depression, the signs and causes, where to find help and support are covered. There is a section giving advice for friends and relatives and some references for further reading.
Contact Mind (see Appendix 1).

Understanding seasonal affective disorder
Describes SAD, its symptoms, causes and the people most likely to suffer from it. It describes how treatment may help SAD. There are details of self-help organisations and references for further reading. This is also available on the internet.
Contact Mind (see Appendix 1).

Index

Have you found **Beating Depression – the 'at your fingertips' guide** practical and useful? If so, you may be interested in other books from Class Publishing.

Positive Action for Health and Wellbeing – Progress Kit
NEW!   £29.99 including VAT
Using straightforward, easy and effective methods, Dr Roet shows you tried and tested steps to better health and self esteem. In his complete programme, Dr Roet reinforces the practical messages in the book with a comprehensive double cassette pack, and personal progress diary.

Parkinson's: a patient's view
Sidney Dorros   £19.99
Parkinson's: a patient's view is a deeply moving account of one man's experiences in coming to terms with life with Parkinson's disease. Sidney Dorros describes, with honesty and courage, how he dealt with Parkinson's for more than 20 years and learned to achieve 'accommodation without surrender'.

Dementia: Alzheimer's and other dementias – the 'at your fingertips' guide
NEW SECOND EDITION!   £14.99
Harry Cayton, Dr Nori Graham and Dr James Warner
At last – a book that tells you everything you need to know about Alzheimer's and other dementias.

'An invaluable contribution to understanding all forms of dementia.'
Dr Jonathan Miller CBE, President of the Alzheimer's Disease Society

Stroke – the 'at your fingertips' guide
Dr Anthony Rudd, Penny Irwin SRN and Bridget Penhale   £14.99
This essential guidebook tells you all about strokes – most importantly how to recover from them. It is full of practical advice, and includes recuperation plans; you will find this book invaluable.

Stop that heart attack!
NEW SECOND EDITION!   £14.99
Dr Derrick Cutting
The easy, drug-free and medically accurate way to cut your risk of having a heart attack dramatically. Even if you already have heart disease, you can halt and even reverse its progress by following Dr Cutting's simple steps. Don't be a victim – take action NOW!

Multiple sclerosis – the 'at your fingertips' guide
Ian Robinson, Dr Stuart Neilson and Dr Frank Clifford   £14.99
Straightforward and positive answers to all your questions about MS.

'An invaluable resource.'
Jan Hatch, MS Society

High blood pressure – the 'at your fingertips' guide
NEW SECOND EDITION!   £14.99
Dr Julian Tudor Hart with Dr Tom Fahey
The authors use all their years of experience as blood pressure experts to answer your questions on high blood pressure.

'Readable and comprehensive information.'
Dr Sylvia McLaughlan, Director General, The Stroke Association

Heart health – the 'at your fingertips' guide
NEW SECOND EDITION!   £14.99
Dr Graham Jackson
This practical handbook, written by a leading cardiologist, answers all your questions about heart conditions.

'Contains the answers the doctor wishes he had given if only he'd had the time.'
Dr Thomas Stuttaford, The Times

PRIORITY ORDER FORM

Cut out or photocopy this form and send it (post free in the UK) to:

Class Publishing Priority Service   **Tel: 01752 202301**
FREEPOST (PAM 6219)   **Fax: 01752 202333**
Plymouth PL6 7ZZ

Please send me urgently   *Post included*
(*tick boxes below*)   *price per copy (UK only)*

☐ **Beating depression – the 'at your fingertips' guide**   £17.99
    (ISBN 1 859590 63 2)

☐ **Positive action for health and wellbeing – progress kit**   £32.99
    (ISBN 1 859590 41 1)

☐ **Parkinson's: a patient's view**   £22.99
    (ISBN 1 872362 70 2)

☐ **Dementia: Alzheimer's and other dementias**
    – the 'at your fingertips' guide   £17.99
    (ISBN 1 872362 91 5)

☐ **Stroke – the 'at your fingertips' guide**   £17.99
    (ISBN 1872362 98 2)

☐ **Stop that heart attack!**   £17.99
    (ISBN 1 859590 55 1)

☐ **Multiple sclerosis – the 'at your fingertips' guide**   £17.99
    (ISBN 1 872362 94 X)

☐ **High blood pressure – the 'at your fingertips' guide**   £17.99
    (ISBN 1 872362 81 8)

☐ **Heart health – the 'at your fingertips' guide**   £17.99
    (ISBN 1 859590 09 8)

                                    TOTAL _____

Easy ways to pay

Cheque: I enclose a cheque payable to Class Publishing for £ _____

Credit card: Please debit my ☐ Access ☐ Visa ☐ Amex ☐ Switch

Number _____ Expiry date _____

Name _____

My address for delivery is _____

_____

Town _____ County _____ Postcode _____

Telephone number (in case of query) _____

Credit card billing address if different from above _____

_____

Town _____ County _____ Postcode _____

Class Publishing's guarantee: remember that if, for any reason, you are not satisfied with these books, we will refund all your money, without any questions asked. Prices and VAT rates may be altered for reasons beyond our control.